Central Visual Field Defects in Glaucoma

Tutul Chakravarti

ISBN 978-90-6299-334-5

Standard soft cover print-on-demand edition. See our website for premium editions of our books.

Kugler Publications
P.O. Box 20538
1001 NM Amsterdam, The Netherlands
www.kuglerpublications.com

Kugler Publications is an imprint of SPB Academic Publishing bv, P.O. Box 20538, 1001 NM Amsterdam, The Netherlands

Table of Contents

List of abbreviations

CC: Cluster Criteria
CMVFD: central-most visual field defect
cpRNFL: circumpapillary retinal nerve fiber layer
CVFD: central visual field defect
GHT: Glaucoma Hemifield Test
HFA: Humphrey Field Analyzer
HRT: Heidelberg Retina Tomograph
HTG: high-tension glaucoma
INS: initial nasal step
IOP: intraocular pressure
IPFS: initial parafoveal scotoma
IPL: inner plexiform layer
IVZ: inferior vulnerability zone
mGCIPL: macular ganglion cell-inner plexiform layer
MD: Mean Deviation
MRA: Moorfields Regression Analysis
MVZ: macular vulnerability zone
NTG: normal-tension glaucoma
OCT: optical coherence tomography
OHTS: Ocular Hypertension Treatment Study
ONH: optic nerve head
PD: Pattern Deviation
PFS: parafoveal scotoma
PNS: paranasal scotoma
POAG: primary open-angle glaucoma
PSD: Pattern Standard Deviation
QoL: quality of life
RGC: retinal ganglion cell
RNFL: retinal nerve fiber layer
SAP: standard automated perimetry
SVZ: superior vulnerability zone
TD: Total Deviation
VF: visual field
VFI: Visual Field Index

Foreword

Glaucoma affects almost 100 million individuals worldwide and it is the leading cause of irreversible blindness. More than half of such individuals are undiagnosed; in some areas of the world, this figure climbs to more than 80% of individuals who go undiagnosed and are unaware they have glaucoma. Ten million individuals are blind in at least 1 eye from glaucoma. So many more individuals have impairment of vision that impact their performance of daily activities. In part, this stems from the failure to 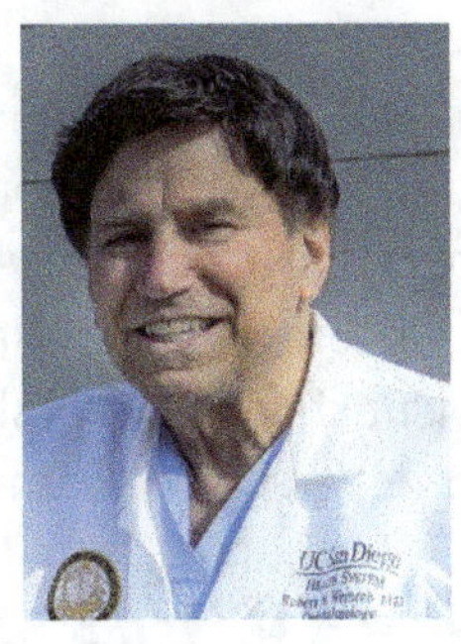 diagnose as well as the failure to detect disease worsening in patients with existing glaucoma. With earlier diagnosis and detection, it is presumed that more timely management would reduce disease worsening and possible blindness. So how will a knowledge of central visual filed defects make a difference and lead to improved diagnosis and management?

Despite improvements in imaging and their interpretation, detection of visual field abnormalities remains the most widely used method for diagnosing and monitoring glaucoma. Although glaucomatous visual field defects can occur throughout the entire visual field, they are typically only tested within the central 24° or 30°. However, central visual field defects often are detected before peripheral ones. And for patients with existing glaucoma, a central visual field defect will often demonstrate worsening prior to a peripheral one. Thus, it follows that testing of the central visual field should be an essential part of glaucoma evaluation.

Despite a formidable body of research demonstrating the importance of testing the central visual field for glaucoma evaluation, it is often omitted by clinicians. However, this practice needs to change. With a clear exposition of the accumulated knowledge of central visual field defects and their testing, Tutul Chakravarti provides the background for stimulating its use by clinicians everywhere. Her explanations of the rationale for central visual field testing are thorough. Moreover, throughout the book she provides practical examples of its application that should resonate with all clinicians caring for glaucoma patients. Surely, this is a book that should be read by all such clinicians!

Despite the imminent emergence of novel testing methods (*e.g.,* virtual perimetry,) and analytics (*e.g.,* deep learning strategies) for visual field testing, it seems certain that the foundational importance of testing of the central visual field will endure. If not already done, therefore, central visual field testing should be implemented without delay into one's clinical practice for glaucoma management!

Robert N. Weinreb, MD
Director, Shiley Eye Institute
Distinguished Professor and Chair of Ophthalmology
Distinguished Professor of Bioengineering
Morris Gleich MD Chair of Glaucoma
Director, Hamilton Glaucoma Center
University of California San Diego

Foreword

We are very pleased to coauthor a foreword for this new book by Dr. Tutul Chakravarti. By way of introduction, the 2 of us began collaborating nearly 30 years ago when we worked together on the development of the original SITA testing algorithms used in the Humphrey perimeter. Over the years, we also have toured much of South Asia together, lecturing on the use of perimetry in glaucoma management, becoming close friends in the process.

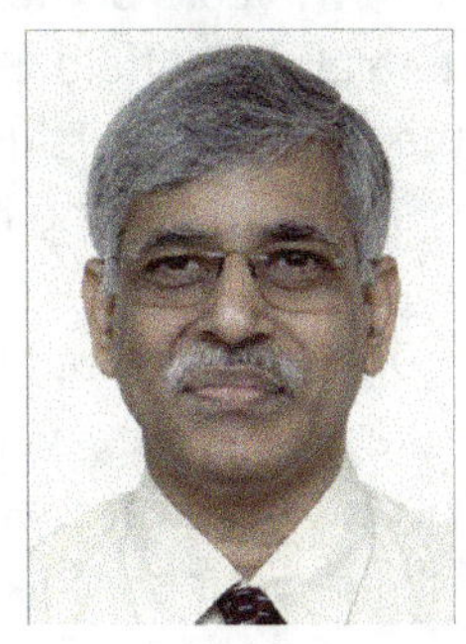

When we were trained, glaucomatous central visual field loss (known to some in those days as macular field loss), was generally considered to be something that was mostly encountered in advanced glaucoma. To be sure, Aulhorn, Drance, Heijl, and others recognised long ago that central visual field damage also happens in early and moderate glaucoma, but it was not acknowledged as a common or compelling issue. In recent years, we all have recognised its importance, but even today we continue to struggle with how best to detect and manage glaucomatous central field loss in daily clinical care.

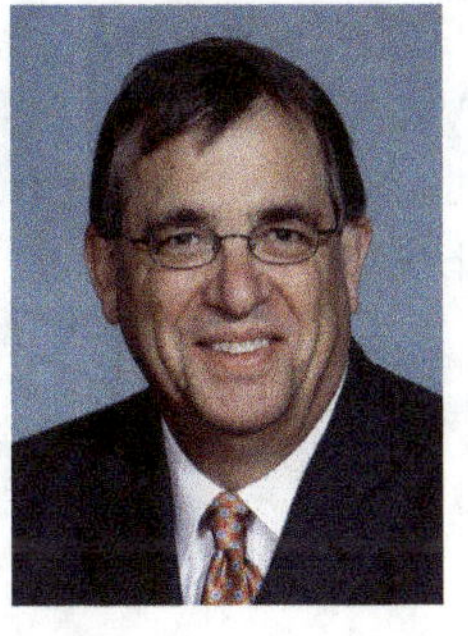

Dr. Tutul Chakravarti is an Indian glaucoma specialist who trained in 4 separate fellowship programs, 2 in Europe and 2 in North America. With this book, we believe that she has distinguished herself as a strong leader in our profession. In *Central Visual Field Defects in Glaucoma*, Dr. Chakravarti has summarised the relevant literature on glaucomatous central field loss and has organised it in wonderfully helpful ways. Although each of us could perform our own literature review of this important topic, Dr. Chakravarti has very generously saved us the trouble. We also realise that authors reviewing this topic for a peer-reviewed journal might not be allowed to cover the literature as completely as she has been able to do throughout the course of this textbook.

Central Visual Field Defects in Glaucoma will not only help us all make sense of many years of international discussions regarding detailed testing of the central visual field, it will also serve as a very helpful reference when clinical questions arise. Thus, we find this new contribution to be quite appropriate at the moment and heartily recommend it to all eye care specialists.

Dr. Chakravarti, thank you for stepping forward to create this new book. Today, there are very few perimetry books that are up to date with the current literature, and clearly your contribution is completely current. We will use your book, and we urge all our colleagues to do so as well.

G. Chandra Sekhar, MD
Vice Chair, Emeritus
LV Prasad Eye Institute
Hyderabad, India

Vincent Michael Patella, OD
Department of Ophthalmology
University of Iowa
Iowa City, IA, USA

Preface

"Tamasa ma jyotirgamaya" / "Lead me from darkness to light"

Brihadaranyaka Upanishad 1.3.8
circa 7th-6th BCE Sanskrit philosophical text

Glaucoma is a leading cause of irreversible blindness, making early detection and management crucial. Protecting central vision is the ultimate goal of glaucoma treatment, yet common visual field tests often overlook early signs of central visual field defects (CVFDs), which can significantly impact the quality of life for glaucoma patients. This book offers a comprehensive guide to understanding CVFDs at all stages of glaucoma, from early detection to advanced cases, providing cutting-edge insights into the detection, diagnosis, and management of CVFDs gleaned from the latest scientific data as well as clinical practice.

Poor detection and underrating of central defects and their progression may cause severe vision loss, even in patients with suspected or early glaucoma, which affects the quality of care from the outset of disease. Hence, the detection of CVFDs is essential in the diagnosis and management of glaucoma even at the earliest stages. There are no accepted standard guidelines for detecting progression in advanced glaucoma with central defects. Therefore, a better understanding of the patterns of CVFDs and their development over time is crucial to improve the management of glaucoma.

This book is primarily written for the use of practicing ophthalmologists and optometrists as well as young trainees in these disciplines who will be at the forefront of glaucoma care in the near future. Eye care specialists who seek an overview of the basic principles may choose to read the first 4 chapters of this book to understand CVFDs in glaucoma. The first 2 chapters lay the foundation for understanding the types of glaucomatous visual field defects and comprehending CVFDs in early glaucoma. Chapter 1 presents one of the most difficult subjects in glaucoma for all ophthalmologists: classification of visual field abnormalities in highly myopic eyes without pathological change. Underlining the relationship between retinal ganglion cell loss and visual field loss varies depending on the stage of the disease, Chapter 3 focuses on the structural techniques and functional tests employed to diagnose glaucoma. The combination of optical coherence tomography and visual field testing is beneficial for disease monitoring, as it allows more frequent detection of disease progression than using either method alone. The chapter then zooms into the evaluation of the structure-function correlation of the 24-2 and 10-2 visual field tests with macular ganglion cell layer/inner plexiform layer thickness, explaining the most salient concepts with schematic models and specifying the relative vulnerability zones of the optic disc to early glaucomatous damage. Chapter 4 discusses the limitations of the 24-2 visual field test to adequately estimate central visual field damage in the early stages of glaucoma.

Current glaucoma staging systems to measure the disease severity are discussed in Chapter 5, which makes it an ideal primer for young trainees in residency and optometric training programs.

Chapter 6 attempts to solve the riddle of whether glaucomatous CVFDs can be evaluated by both 24-2 and 10-2 tests as well as the utility of 10-2 tests for evaluating CVFDs in early glaucoma. The long-term debate about whether 10-2 testing detects any additional defects not identified in 24-2 testing is central to this chapter, which explores two questions. How and why would a 10-2 visual field test pattern be a better instrument for recognizing CVFDs? Does the 10-2 visual field test provide sufficient additional information to the 24-2 visual field test to warrant its routine use in the evaluation and management of early-stage glaucoma? Chapter 7 touches upon how the severity of central damage can be assessed and predicted by these two tests (24-2 and 10-2) and provides a point-based analysis of the visual field in addition to the factors related to abnormal 24-2 visual field points responsible for the presence of parafoveal scotomas on the 10-2 visual field. The chapter in question is integral to Chapter 6 and as companion chapters, they will hopefully guide clinicians to successfully predict the severity of CVFDs.

Chapters 8 to 10 navigate established and novel methods of evaluating the visual field to detect glaucomatous damage. In routine clinical practice, using a single test to evaluate both the central 10° area and the total 30° visual field simultaneously for detecting glaucomatous damage is a useful tool. The scope of testing the central and peripheral visual field separately is limited as it demands extra time and cost. In this respect, is the new 24-2C a better choice to end these debates, or is the Octopus G1 program the only solution? Another burning and controversial issue is whether the 24-2C test strategies—with extra central test locations—included in the new Humphrey Field Analyzer 3 (ZEISS) show enhanced ability to improve the detection of central defects over the standard 24-2 visual field.

Is the SITA Faster algorithm a better alternative than the SITA Standard algorithm, even after abandoning the blind spot catch trial and false-negative catch trial? Chapter 9 delves into this issue while also outlining the interpretation of 24-2C test results as well as the evolution of the SITA Faster paradigm and its potential benefits and limitations. Chapter 10 offers a primer on the Octopus perimeter, focusing specifically on the detection and interpretation of CVFDs by means of its G1 program.

Chapter 11 contains an in-depth discussion regarding the modes and methods of characterizing and classifying central visual field loss in advanced glaucoma. Crucial factors such as how to evaluate disease progression in advanced-stage glaucoma on the 24-2 and 10-2 visual field tests, the characterization and classification of central visual field loss in advanced glaucoma, central visual field loss patterns and their shifts in advanced glaucoma, and the impact of filtration surgery on CVFDs in advanced glaucoma complete the book's final chapter.

On a personal note, I especially wish to recognize my year-long (2019–2020) Fulbright-Nehru Academic and Professional Excellence Fellowship at the Hamilton Glaucoma Center, University of California San Diego, CA, United States, for enabling me to study CVFDs in glaucoma. It was a rare privilege for me to have interacted with stalwarts in the field during this Fellowship period. I wish to thank my host faculty, Professor Linda M. Zangwill (Professor of Ophthalmology, Co-Director of Clinical Research, and Director of the IDEA at the Hamilton Glaucoma Center), who helped me immensely in understanding this subject.

It is difficult to adequately express my gratitude to Professor Robert N. Weinreb (Chair and Distinguished Professor of Ophthalmology, Director of the Shiley Eye Institute, and Director of the Hamilton Glaucoma Center), who not only always answered my queries, however insignificant, and inspired me to probe and think about the questions raised in this book, but also took the time to read the book before print and write a compelling foreword. I would also like to extend my deepest appreciation to G. Chandra Sekhar, MD (Vice Chair Emeritus at the LV Prasad Eye Institute in Hyderabad, India) and Vincent Michael Patella, OD (Department of Ophthalmology, University of Iowa, IA, USA), two luminaries and long-time advocates of this book's topic for their thoughtful contribution in their jointly written foreword. This book would not have been possible without guidance from Professor George L. Spaeth, Director Emeritus of Glaucoma Service at Wills Eye Hospital (Philadelphia, PA, USA), who first opened my eyes to the world of glaucoma research in 2006 while I was a Glaucoma Research Fellow at Wills Eye Hospital.

I record my most sincere thanks to Kugler Publications, and particularly Mr. Simon Bakker, its Managing Director, for kindly publishing my manuscript. I would like to express my sincere gratitude to Ms. Silvia Sanchez Di Martino of Kugler Publications, who considerably helped improving the manuscript.

Dr. Tutul Chakravarti, *MBBS, DO, DNB*
Eye and Glaucoma Care, Kolkata, India
January 2025

About the author

Dr. Tutul Chakravarti, MBBS, DO, DNB, is an Indian ophthalmologist specializing in glaucoma who has been engaged in sustained clinical research since 2006.

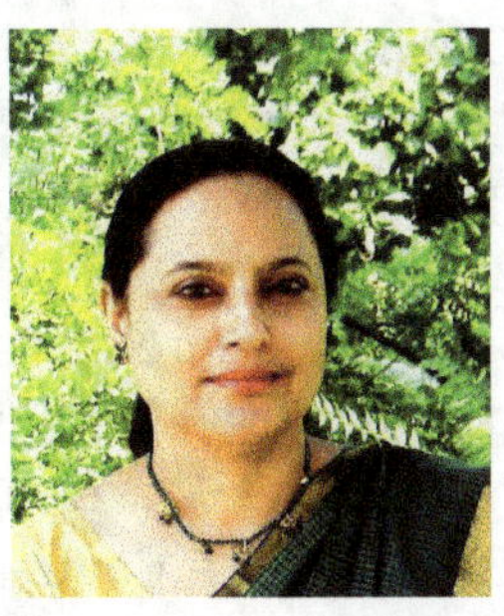

She received the International Council of Ophthalmology Research Fellowship Award in neuro-ophthalmology at Imperial College, London in 2005. The following year she completed her glaucoma research fellowship at Wills Eye Hospital, Philadelphia, United States, under the supervision of Professor George L. Spaeth, moving onto a second glaucoma research fellowship at Rotterdam Eye Hospital, The Netherlands in 2009.

In 2014, she earned a Postgraduate Diploma in Epidemiology from the Indian Institute of Public Health in New Delhi. Dr. Chakravarti was awarded the prestigious research grant from the Indian Government's Department of Science and Technology as the principal investigator for the project "Assessment of glaucomatous damage and its socioeconomic impacts in West Bengal", conducted from 2014 to 2017.

She was awarded the Fulbright-Nehru Academic and Professional Excellence Fellowship (2019–2020) and affiliated to the Hamilton Glaucoma Center at the Shiley Eye Institute, University of California San Diego, United States, for her project on Developing a Disease Severity Scoring System for Patients with Primary-Open Angle Glaucoma. She has been awarded International Ophthalmic Heroes of India Award by the All India Ophthalmological Society at the 2022 and 2024 AIOC Annual Conferences.

Dr. Chakravarti served in premier medical institutions in Delhi and Calcutta as a glaucoma specialist and as an anterior segment surgeon. She has also contributed to postgraduate teaching in ophthalmology in a teaching hospital affiliated to the University of Calcutta as an Associate Professor.

A member of the national faculty of the Glaucoma Society of India since 2012, Dr. Chakravarti has also been inducted as a Member of the Patient Committee of the World Glaucoma Association in 2022. She is the Founder-Secretary of Eye & Glaucoma Care, a trust dedicated to caring for glaucoma patients, in Kolkata, India.

She has more than twenty research papers on glaucoma to her credit in peer-reviewed journals as first and corresponding author. Her publication "Agreement Between 10-2 and 24-2C Visual Field Test Protocols for Detecting Glaucomatous Central Visual Field Defects" was considered the Paper of the Month by the Advisory Board of the World Glaucoma Association in June 2021. Dr. Chakravarti also published one of the first studies comparing the Humphrey Field Analyzer 24-2C program to the 10-2 to detect central visual field loss.

Chapter 1

Types of glaucomatous visual field defects

This chapter describes the types of glaucomatous VF defects and their characteristics with an emphasis on glaucomatous central visual field defects (CVFDs) located within the central 10° of the 24-2 or 30-2 VF.

1. Perimetry is essential for diagnosing and managing glaucoma

For glaucoma patients, VF testing identifies the presence of any glaucomatous damage and quantifies the amount of VF loss. Reproducible VF defects demonstrated by test results are the most definite means of confirming a diagnosis of chronic open-angle glaucoma. VF testing provides a unique insight into the impact of glaucoma on the individual since it combines the information on the detection with that on the location of VF defects.

2. A broad understanding of central, mid-peripheral, and peripheral VF defects

Glaucomatous VF defects occur throughout the field of vision, including the central 10°, the mid-periphery (as measured in standard tests over the central 24°–30°), and the far periphery. However, they are most frequently tested over the central 24°–30° of vision. Far peripheral testing is seldom used in routine clinical assessment of glaucoma, although previous studies suggest that it provides relevant information independent of that gained from central testing.

3. Typical VF defects in glaucoma

In clinical practice for differentiating between normal and glaucomatous eyes, the 24-2 size III white SITA Standard threshold test of the HFA (Carl Zeiss Meditec, Dublin, CA, USA) is one of the most frequently used tests and considered the best choice for this purpose. Glaucoma is a disease resulting in the degeneration of retinal nerve fiber bundles in the eye. Since the largest proportion of retinal nerve fibers is located within the central 30°, most early to moderate glaucoma VF defects occur within the central 30°. Typical defect patterns follow the distribution of the retinal nerve fiber bundles and there is a clear separation along the superior and inferior hemifields at the horizontal meridian (Figs. 1-1, 1-2).

The OHTS (2003) provides a classification for characterizing different types of glaucomatous VF defects.[1] The typical patterns of VF loss on account of glaucoma are arcuate, partial arcuate, paracentral, nasal step, temporal wedge, and altitudinal damage (Fig. 1-3). OHTS observed that the most frequent glaucomatous VF defects were partial arcuate, paracentral, and nasal step defects.[1] Due to its high reproducibility, the OHTS classification system has been widely accepted for clinical practice and research for recognizing VF abnormalities. However, several different types of defects often occur concurrently in the same field.

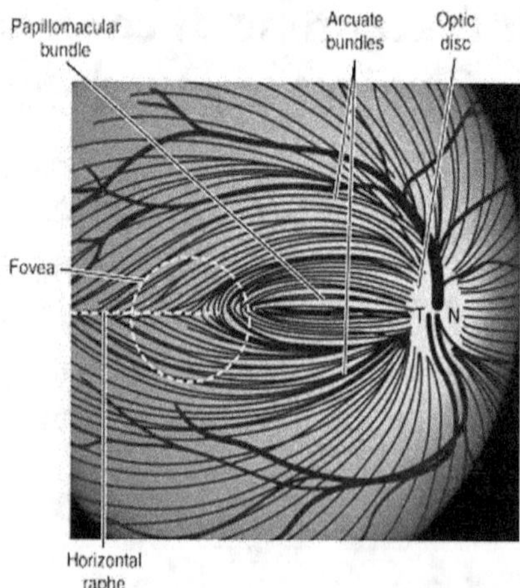

Fig. 1-1. Retinal nerve fibers enter the optic disc in a specific manner. The arrangement of nerve fibers in the optic disc corresponds to their pattern of arrival from the retina. Reproduced from Balcer and Prasad.[2]

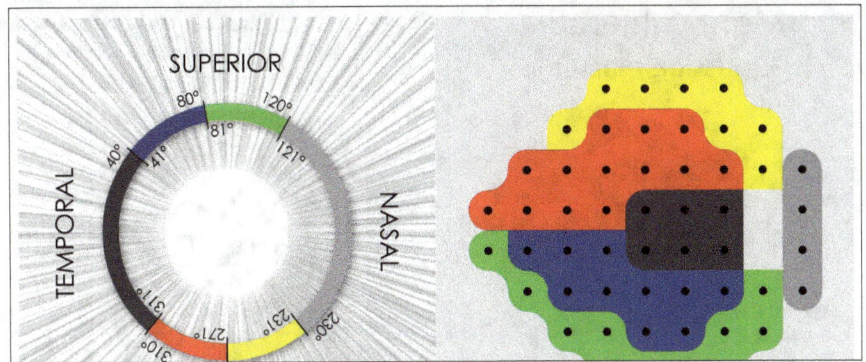

Fig. 1-2. Map representing the relationship between SAP VF sectors and sections of the peripapillary OCT scan circle. **(Right)** Yellow corresponds to Superior/Nasal; red corresponds to Superior/Temporal; blue corresponds to Inferior/Temporal; and green corresponds to Inferior/Nasal. Reproduced from Bizios *et al.*[3]

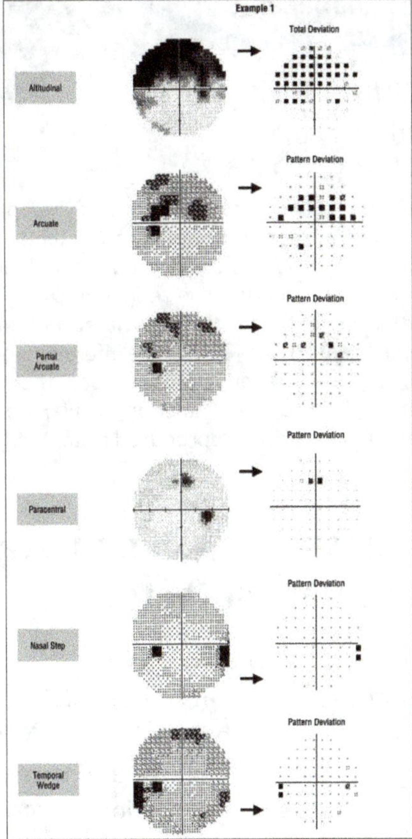

Fig. 1-3. Examples of classifications of VF abnormalities from the OHTS study.[1] Typical patterns of VF loss on account of glaucoma are arcuate, partial arcuate, paracentral, nasal step, temporal wedge, and altitudinal damage. Reproduced from Keltner *et al.*[1]

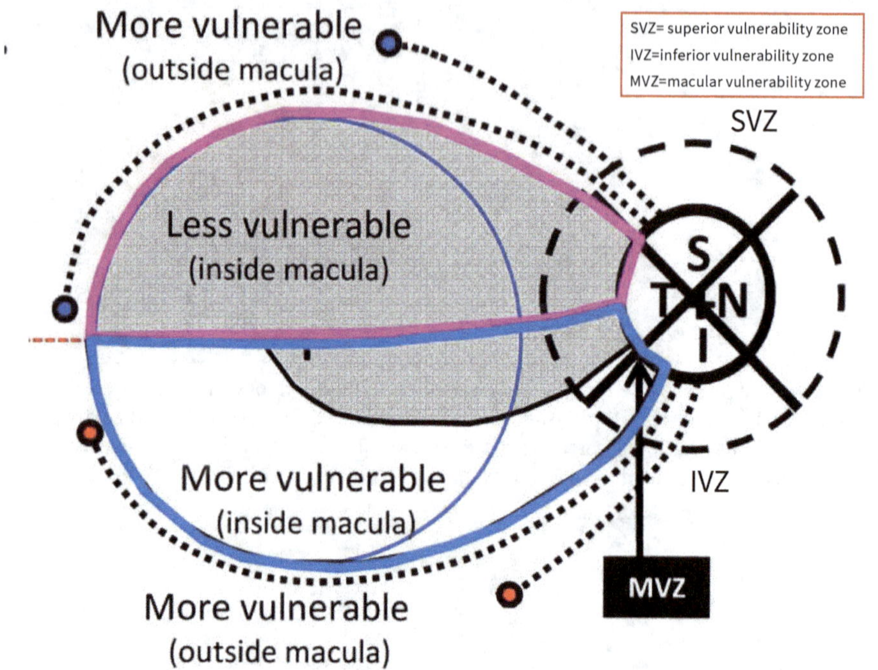

Fig. 1-4. The schematic model illustrates the regions of the optic disc most vulnerable to local glaucomatous damage as reported by Hood.[4] The temporal half of the disc has 2 vulnerable regions: the SVZ and the IVZ. The MVZ is one part of the IVZ, encompassing the inferotemporal section of the optic nerve. The retinal areas most vulnerable to glaucomatous damage include the area of the macula associated with the MVZ (the white region within the light blue borders). Most of the RGCs of the inferior macula project mostly to the inferior quadrant of the disc. The RGC axons from the rest of the macula (maculo-papillary region of the inferior macula plus the entire superior macula) project to the relatively less vulnerable temporal quadrant of the disc. Reproduced from Hood.[4]

4. Recent understanding of non-standard and non-conventional VF defects

A recent understanding of a wide variety of VF defects is available based on the improved concept of cpRNFL damage on OCT. Several investigators have identified the regions of the optic disc most vulnerable to local glaucomatous damage and detected an SVZ, an IVZ, and a MVZ (Fig. 1-4).[4-6] Because of variations of cpRNFL defects, wide variation in the depth, width, and homogeneity of the RNFL damage is expected in the MVZ, SVZ, and IVZ.[4] Due to these variant cpRNFL defects, some VF damage types do not fall into the conventional VF defect classification. While some VF defects of those varieties perfectly match the classic pattern of VF defects described by the OHTS classification, some may not correspond to the classic pattern.[4] There is relatively less discussion of non-conventional VF defects in the literature. For example, CVFD is relatively poorly discussed despite its potential implication of causing a greater decrease in vision-related quality of life, even in the early disease stage.

OHTS classified CVFD as "other patterns of VF loss". As per OHTS classification, CVFD is likely to be due to ocular or neurologic abnormalities other than glaucoma. However, it is not surprising that non-standard and non-conventional VF defects are relatively more common than previously expected. The MVZ, SVZ, and IVZ regions are described in detail in Chapter 3.

5. The CVFD in glaucoma

Damage to the immediate paracentral VF, resulting in the so-called split fixation, which as per the common assumption, is a sign of advanced loss in cases of end-stage glaucoma (Fig. 1-5).[7] Evidence lately available, however, may indicate that central visual defect is a feature, characteristic not just merely of the late stages or end stage of glaucoma, but also of its earliest stages (Fig. 1-6).[8] It has been recognized over a long period that glaucomatous damage can affect the central field and macula (*e.g.*, Aulhorn and Harms, 1967;[9] Drance, 1969;[10] Heijl and Lundqvist, 1984[11]). It is therefore likely that central VF defects could be a clinical feature in the early stage of the disease.[12,13] Glaucomatous VF loss can affect the immediate paracentral area, particularly the upper hemifield, which may be noted even in eyes with mild to moderate glaucoma.[14]

A 24-2 VF **B** 10-2 VF

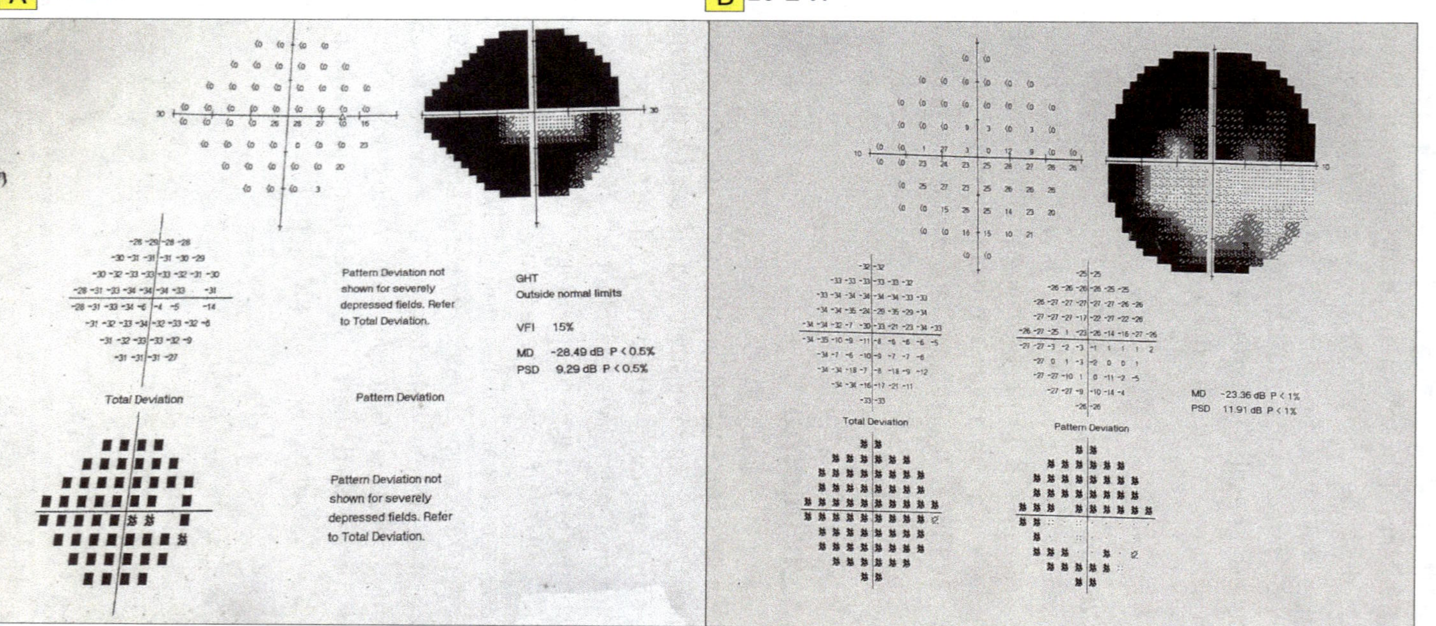

Fig. 1-5. A patient with POAG with advanced VF loss in his right eye in 24-2 and 10-2 tests. **(A)** Advanced VF loss in a case of end-stage glaucoma on a 24-2 visual field test where the central island of vision remains only in the inferior hemifield. This VF test shows a VFI of 15%, MD of -28.49 dB, and PSD of 9.29 dB. **(B)** The central 10-2 pattern is useful for following the progression of this patient with advanced VF loss on a 24-2 VF test pattern. The MD is -23.36 dB and PSD is 11.91 dB on the 10-2 VF test.

Initial VF defect on 24-2 VF

VF defect on 24-2 VF after 3 years

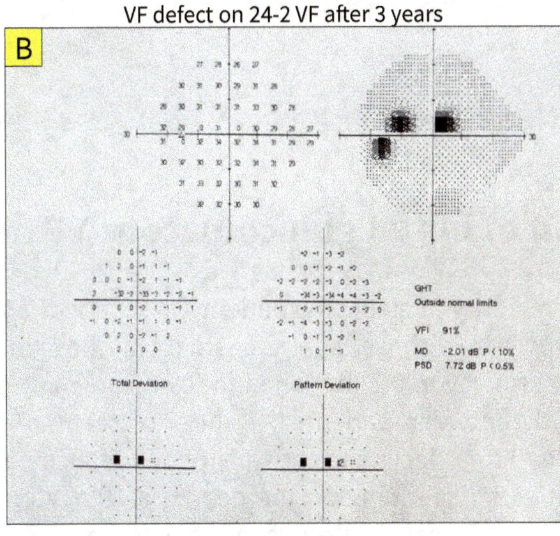

Fig. 1-6. The earliest glaucomatous defect was documented as a central VF defect in 24-2 and 10-2 VF tests. **(A)** This VF documents the earliest glaucomatous defect of a POAG patient as a single abnormal 24-2 VF test point located in the superior nasal hemifield within the central 5° in his left eye. This 24-2 VF had an MD of -0.44 dB and PSD of 2.65 dB; the GHT interpreted this VF as Outside Normal Limits. The single abnormal point was present in both the TD and PD probability plots. **(B)** After 3 years this patient presented with a typical parafoveal scotoma in the superior hemifield in 24-2 VF with much worse MD (-2.01 dB) and PSD (7.72 dB) than the initial VF loss in (A). **(C)** The same patient was tested with a 10-2 test pattern and the severity of the central VF defect was more evident as an arcuate defect in the 10-2 VF test pattern. It is interesting to note that the MD (-6.02 dB) and PSD (10.90 dB) were much worse on the 10-2 VF test than the 24-2 VF test.

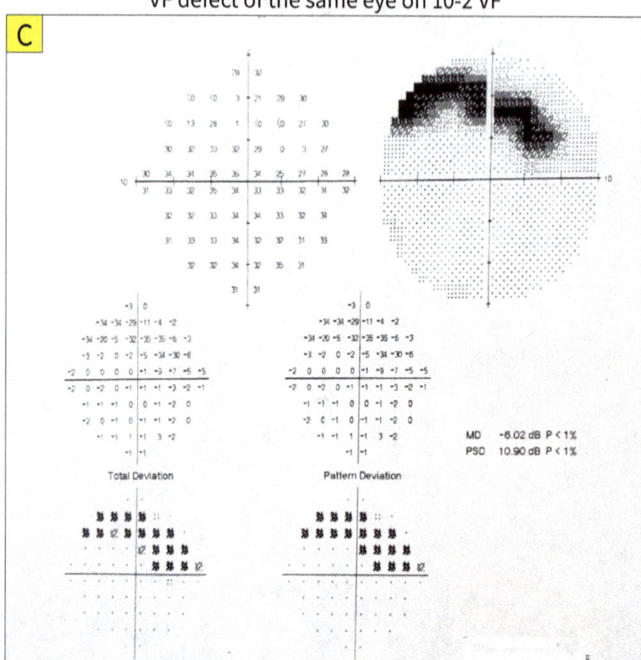

Fig. 1-6. Continued.

6. Location of initial glaucomatous VF defects

Initially, in the majority of glaucoma patients, VF changes are localized. As the disease progresses, these focal areas become broader, deeper, and more abundant. However, the rate and mode of worsening of visual fields vary significantly between patients.[15] Failure to treat early to moderate VF loss could lead to a decline in the quality of a glaucoma patient's life, with various effects depending on the degree and location of the initial VF loss.[16,17] VF defects near fixation have a greater impact on the level of function compared with peripheral damage, even at an early stage of glaucoma.[18,19] A few studies have investigated the location of initial glaucomatous VF defects and their modes of deterioration.[8] Some research has evaluated the risk factors associated with an IPFS compared with an INS in glaucoma patients and indicated that the pattern and location of VF loss may be useful to identify different glaucomatous pathogenetic mechanisms.[19]

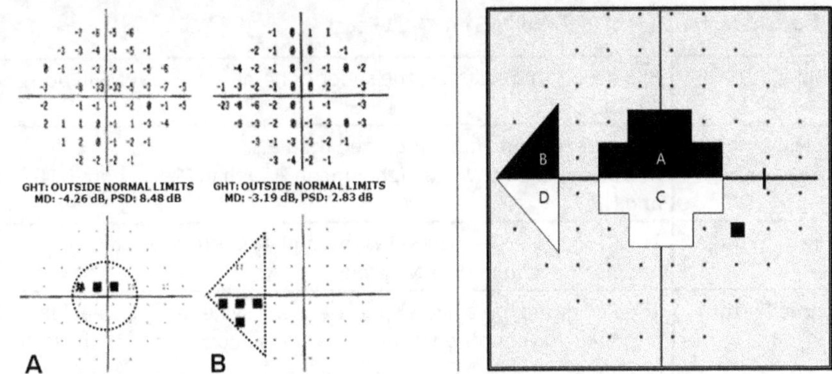

Fig. 1-7. Examples of the 2 patterns of glaucomatous VF defect on the Humphrey 24-2 SITA Standard PD plot are discussed here. **(Left)** The PD is divided into 2 subfields of the Humphrey VF. **(A)** The PFS group includes abnormal points within 12 points of the central 10° radius. **(B)** The PNS group has abnormal points within 12 nasal peripheral points in one hemifield. **(Right)** Location of the initial VF defect. Initial VF defects are divided into 2 groups, paracentral and nasal defects. These 2 groups are further divided into 2 subgroups, superior and inferior, based on the affected hemifield. Reproduced from Park *et al.*[20] and Kim *et al.*[8]

Another study measured the amount and location of ONH abnormal points and the RNFL thickness with paracentral scotomas compared to peripheral scotomas.[8] However, different terminologies have been used to describe central, paracentral, and peripheral VF defects by different research groups, though the basic features are nearly the same in all descriptions. One such instance is "initial parafoveal scotoma (IPFS)", which is almost the same as initial paracentral or central scotoma. Similarly, "peripheral nasal step (PNS)" generally indicates peripheral defect. Chapter 2 discusses the different terminologies in detail.

In the 24-2 test grid, 54 test locations are evenly distributed with a 6° separation. Twelve of the 54 test point locations are in the central 10°. In the 24-2 VF, the PD probability plot can be divided into 2 subfields (PFS and PNS). By definition, the isolated IPFS[20] is located in 1 hemifield of the 24-2 VF within a 10° radius, and the isolated PNS is within the nasal periphery outside 10° of fixation (Fig. 1-7). Table 1-1 and Figure 1-8 describe the characteristic patterns of PFS and PNS. However, in this book, we apply the term CVFD for all defects within the central 10° of the 24-2 VF and we apply the term PNS for any peripheral scotoma or peripheral nasal step.

Table 1-1. Characteristics of PFS and PNS on 24-2 VF test

Location	PFS occurs more often in the superior hemifield than PNS in both NTG and HTG.
Defect severity	PFS is deeper and more localized than PNS. PFS also presents with a higher mean PSD than PNS in both NTG and HPG.
Disc hemorrhage	The PFS group is associated with a higher frequency of disc haemorrhage than the PNS group.
Systemic factors	The PFS group has a higher prevalence of systemic hypotension, migraine, Raynaud's phenomenon, and sleep apnea than the PNS group.
IOP-independent risk factor	PFS may be more associated with IOP-independent risk factors compared with PNS.
Test-retest variability	Point-wise variability in glaucomatous VFs is the lowest in the most central points of the VF than in peripheral points. However, point-wise variability is common at more peripheral points.

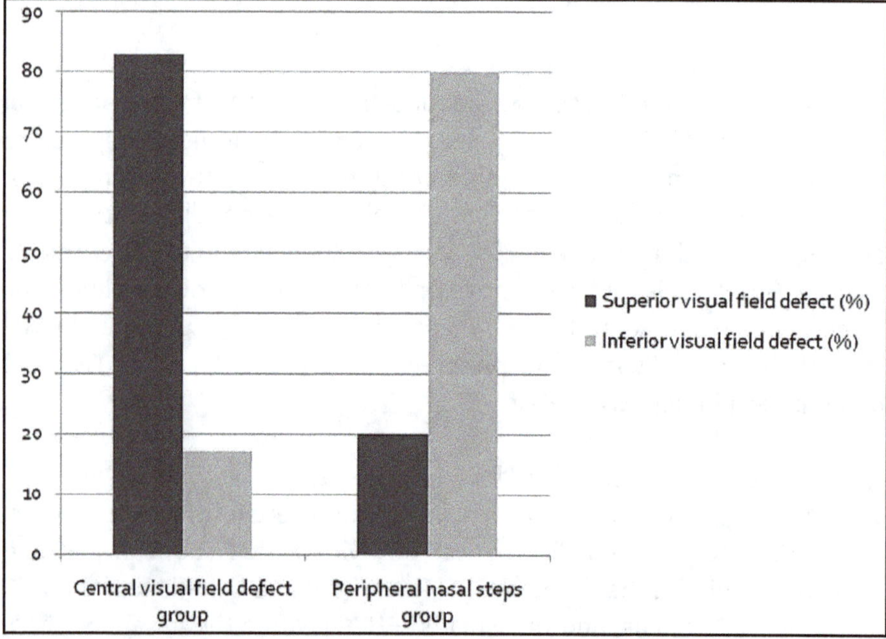

Fig. 1-8. Previous studies have shown that the PFS group on the 24-2 VF test showed a predominance of superior field defects, whereas the PNS group had a higher percentage of inferior field defects. Reproduced from Jung *et al.*[21]

7. VF defects associated with NTG and HTG

The morphology of different VF defects or scotomas in POAG depends on the glaucoma subtype.[22] In NTG, the occurrence of dense scotomas close to fixation is likely to be steeper and more localized at a comparatively early stage in the disease process compared to HTG.[23] However, in chronic simple glaucoma, at the same stage, the occurrence of such defects is less likely.[23] Similar paracentral scotomas tend to occur in association with more advanced field loss in HTG, a subset of POAG. It has been recently reported that NTG patients with PFS have different risk factor profiles; for example, the occurrence of systemic hypotension is higher in patients with PFS compared to those with PNS. The VFI gives greater weight to the centrally located test points than to peripheral points. Hence the VFI value is lower (worse) in the VFs having the PFS group than in the PNS group. However, a PFS does not necessarily mean a loss of functional vision.

8. Optic disc morphology and related PFS

To minimize the progression and loss of vision of glaucoma, early detection and intervention are vital.[24] It has been observed that different patterns of glaucomatous optic disc injury are associated with distinctive pathophysiologic mechanisms. Nicolela and Drance[25,26] classified glaucomatous eyes into 4 optic disc phenotypes based on their appearance. They categorized glaucomatous eyes as focal ischemic, generalized cup enlargement, myopic glaucomatous, and senile sclerotic types. Each phenotype is related to characteristic clinical features. For example, while optic discs with generalized enlargement were related to elevated levels of IOP, optic discs with focal notches were associated with localized VF loss.[27,28]

Similarly, compared to subjects with PNS, subjects with PFS or CVFD show more changes in glaucomatous ONH morphology in the inferior temporal sector,[29] corresponding to superior hemifield defects (Figs. 1-8, 1-9).

Previous research has shown that the optic disc rim in NTG eyes is significantly thinner than in HTG eyes and the largest difference occurs in the inferior and inferotemporal regions. Therefore, at a similar level of VF defect, PFS may involve a greater number of damaged RGCs than PNS.[23]

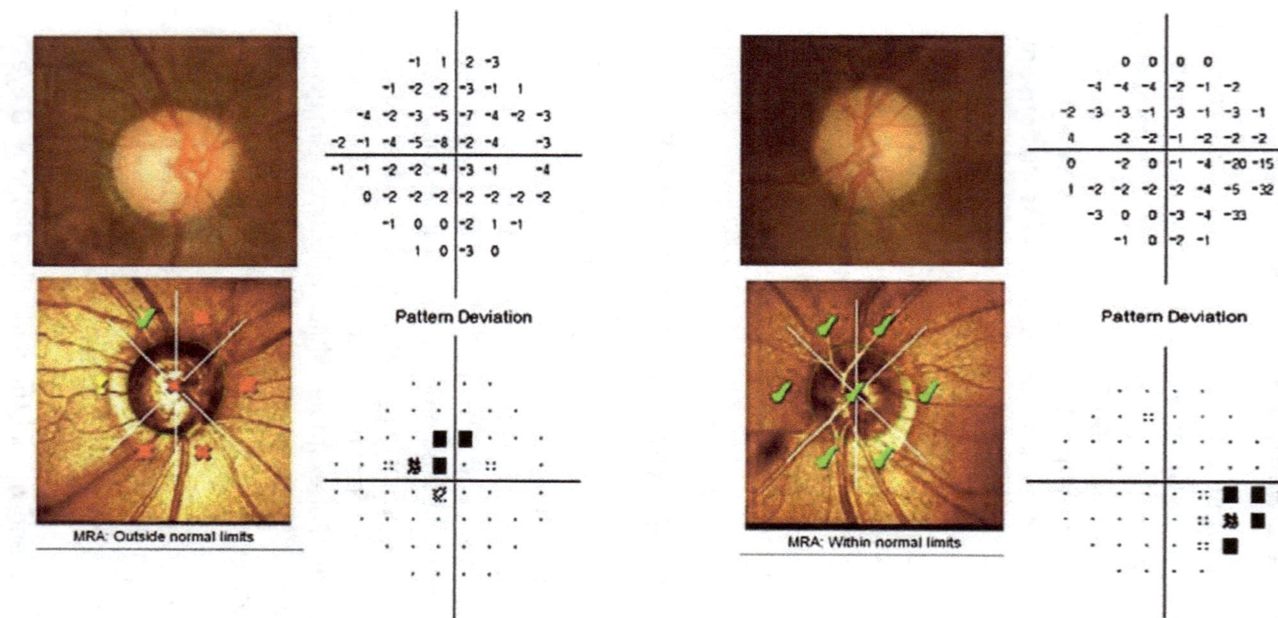

Fig. 1-9. The global and 6-sector (T: temporal; TS: temporal superior; TI: temporal inferior; N: nasal; NS: nasal superior; and NI: nasal inferior) classification of the ONH by HRT's MRA. **(Left)** The eye with superior PFS was classified as outside normal limits by MRA. Sector analysis showed the TI sector to be Outside Normal Limits and the T sector to be Borderline. **(Right)** The eye with the inferior PNS was classified as Within Normal Limits by global and sector analyses of MRA. Reproduced from Jung *et al.*[21]

The PFS group shows a thinner RNFL in the temporal sector, and in the 7 and 8 o'clock sectors, compared to the PNS group. This may explain, at least in part, the predominance of superior VF defects in the PFS group (Fig. 1-8).[21] Global and TI sector on MRA classification by HRT suggested more abnormal optic disc shape in the PFS group in comparison with the PNS group, with a comparable MD and higher PSD (Fig. 1-9).[21]

9. Clinical characteristics of initial superior and inferior PFS

- Superior PFS are generally associated with systemic factors, while inferior PFS are generally associated with ocular factors.
- The superior group has a female preponderance, a higher incidence of disc hemorrhage, and exhibited more association with migraine and less association with hypertension.
- Generally, inferior PFS are more closely associated with ocular factors: steeper and longer axial lengths are associated with inferior defects.

10. Location of initial VF defects in glaucoma and their mode of deterioration

The initial 2 types of VF defects, PFS and PNS, are based on probability map locations in at least 3 out of the initial 4 Humphrey VF printouts.[8] These 2 groups can be further divided into 2 subgroups (superior and inferior) based on the affected hemifield (Fig. 1-7). Horizontally, PFS is limited within points from 0° to 10°, and PNS lies points beyond 20°. Some researchers mentioned them as paracentral defects and nasal defects.

Deterioration of VF defect is defined by modifying the Anderson's criteria. Contiguous points on a Humphrey 24-2 SITA Standard VF with $P < 2\%$ on the TD plot, or any newly developed scotoma (at least 1 point of $P < 1\%$ or 3 contagious points of $P < 2\%$) in the same hemifield, is defined as deterioration.[8] Previous research noted that the direction of worsening of VF defects is either central or peripheral depending on the initial location of the VF defects. To confirm any deterioration of the VF defects at least 3 consecutive VFs are required.[8]

As an example, a case is described here that presents both types of defects at the initial stage of the disease and showing deterioration over 9 years of follow-up (Fig. 1-10). He has superior PFS and PNS on 24-2 VF in the right eye with a history of disc hemorrhage in his right eye.

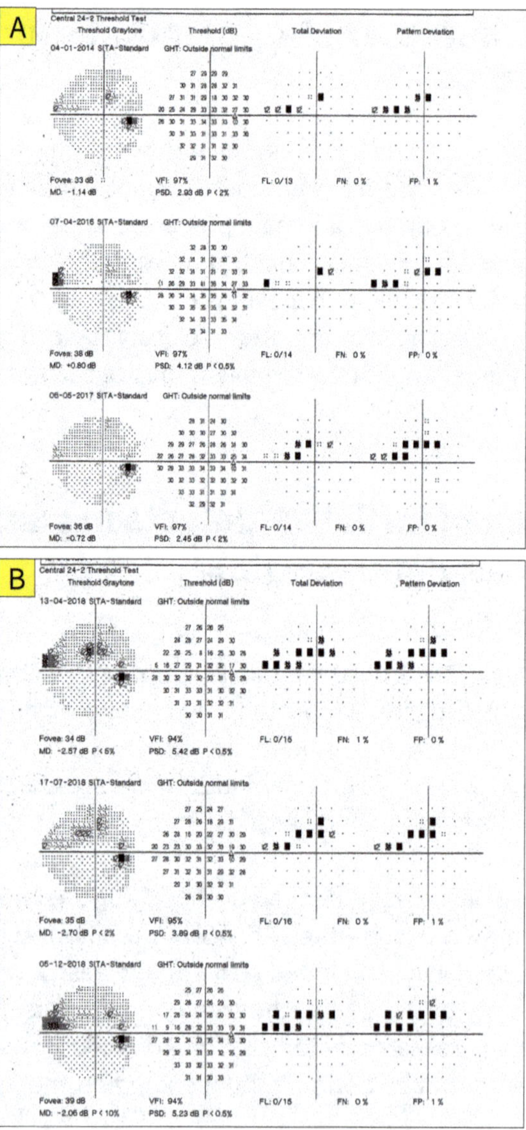

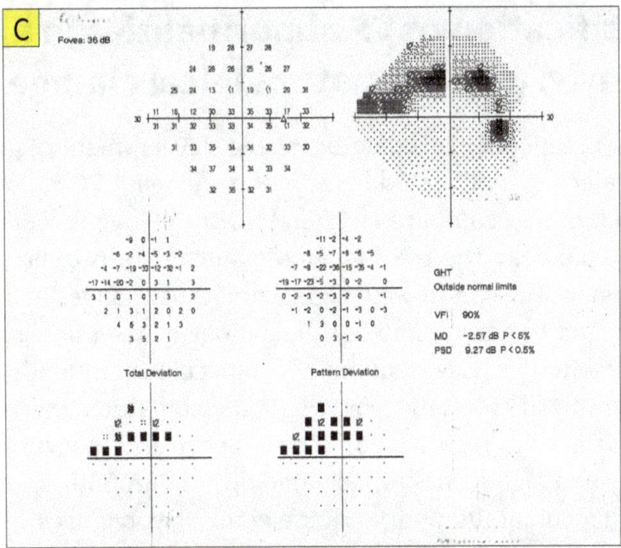

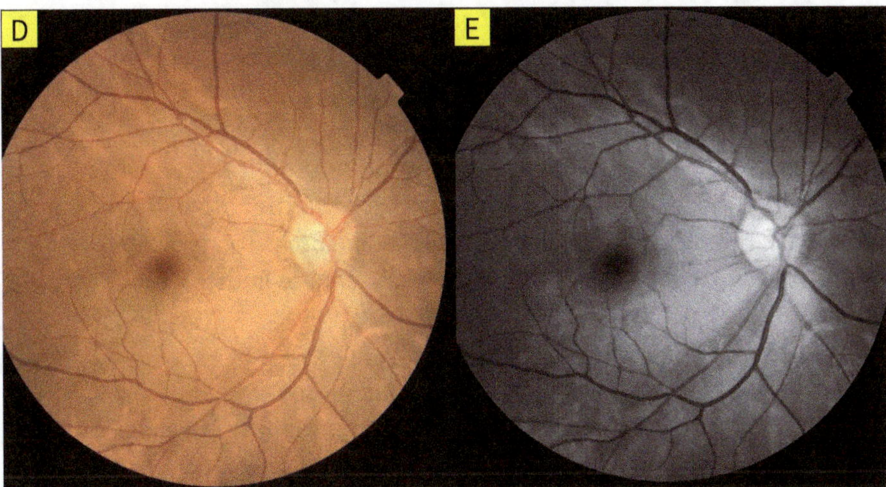

Fig. 1-10. Worsening of initial paracentral and nasal step over the years. This overview of 24-2 VFs present gradual worsening of initial paracentral and nasal step in the upper hemifield of the right eye of a 40-year-old male with NTG. **(A, B)** Overview displaying deteriorating VFs from 2014 to 2018. **(C)** The patient's recent VF defects on 24-2 VF in 2023, which shows an arcuate defect in the upper hemifield with VFI 90%, MD -2.57 MD, and PSD 9.27 dB. **(D)** Fundus photograph of the patient's right eye taken in 2018, which documents glaucomatous inferior RNFL defect with inferior neuroretinal rim narrowing. **(E)** The patient's red-free fundus photograph helps to detect glaucomatous RNFL defects.

11. Classification of VF abnormalities in highly myopic eyes without pathological change

Myopia is an independent risk factor for the development of glaucoma. It has been projected that the odds ratio of developing POAG for eyes with high myopia is 5.9, as compared with eyes without high myopia.[30,31] Again, in highly myopic eyes, the prevalence of glaucomatous optic neuropathy can be as high as 27.2%.[32] However, glaucomatous changes in myopic eyes are often difficult to detect, and ophthalmologists assessing patients with high myopia often face this quandary. Clinicians frequently encounter the challenge of differentiating between glaucomatous and non-glaucomatous VF defects in highly myopic eyes because of concurring myopic maculopathy and high myopia-associated optic neuropathy, both of which can mimic glaucomatous perimetric defects.[33] Myopic eyes may present with typical glaucomatous VF defects or with non-glaucomatous VF defects. Enlarged blind spots are the most frequently observed high myopia-related VF defects in myopic eyes. The frequency of glaucoma-like VF defects is positively associated with older age (OR, 1.07), while the frequency of high myopia-related VF defects is positively associated with longer axial length (OR, 1.65).[34] When myopic patients present with typical glaucomatous VF defects, the diagnosis is relatively straightforward and treatment can be initiated without hesitation. However, when it comes to atypical VF defects associated with uncharacteristic structural changes in the ONH, diagnosing glaucoma in myopic eyes is more challenging.

It is important for clinicians to differentiate between glaucomatous optic nerve damage and non-glaucomatous optic neuropathy because glaucoma can be addressed therapeutically. A recent study proposed a new and reproducible VF classification system that describes VF loss patterns in highly myopic eyes without myopic maculopathy (non-pathologic high myopia).[34]

11.1. The procedure of formulating and assessing the VF classification system

Perimetry is an important tool to diagnose and monitor glaucoma.[35,36] Most pivotal glaucoma studies, such as the Early Manifest Glaucoma Trial, the OHTS, and the United Kingdom Glaucoma Treatment Study, have applied perimetry as the primary endpoint method.[37-39] However, no commonly accepted classification of VF abnormalities in high myopia is available to distinguish between functional damage resulting from glaucoma and damage resulting from high myopia. Therefore, a research group pioneering in the study of high myopia proposed a new and broader VF classification system for highly myopic eyes, based on observation of 1893 VF reports, literature review, and multiple consensus meetings.[34] They observed that 10.8% of highly myopic eyes without myopic maculopathy showed glaucoma-like VF defects, the prevalence of which was associated with longer axial length.[34]

In this VF classification system, first, the 1893 VF test results were categorized based on the OHTS classification, which divides VF defects into nerve fiber bundle abnormalities and non–nerve fiber bundle abnormalities.[30] Next, those VF defects that did not meet any of the definitions of the OHTS classification were considered as novel defect patterns. Lastly, a new classification system for highly myopic eyes was prepared. The classification system comprises 10 VF patterns and 4 major types of VF defects (Table 1-2): normal type, glaucoma-like defects (paracentral defect, nasal step, partial arcuate defect, arcuate defect), high myopia-related defects (enlarged blind spot, vertical step, partial peripheral rim, non-specific defect), and combined defects (nasal step with enlarged blind spot).[34] Examples of the classification of VF abnormalities (with corresponding fundus photographs) are shown in Figure 1-11. Figure 1-12 illustrates the frequency distribution of each VF type in highly myopic eyes. This classification system offers a tool for clinicians to distinguish glaucomatous VF loss from non-glaucomatous VF defects in highly myopic eyes and may also help evaluate the findings of clinical trials and epidemiologic studies.

Table 1-2. Visual field abnormality classification in non-pathologic highly myopic eyes

Type	Pattern	Definition
Normal		Pattern standard deviation within normal limits and no VF defects.*
Glaucoma-like defects	Paracentral detect	A relatively small V detect in the nerve fiber bundle region. The defect generally is not contiguous with the blind spot or the nasal meridian. Does not involve points located outside of 15° that are adjacent to the nasal meridian.
	Nasal step	Limited field loss adjacent to the nasal horizontal meridian. Includes at least 1 abnormal test point** located at or outside of 15° on the nasal horizontal meridian. Can include > 1 abnormal test point in the nerve fiber bundle region on the temporal side. but the abnormal test points on the temporal side cannot be clustered contiguously.
	Partial arcuate defect	VF loss in the nerve fiber bundle region that extends from the temporal side to the nasal side. Must include at least 1 abnormal test point in the temporal half of field. The defect might not be contiguous with either the blind spot or the nasal meridian.
	Arcuate defect	Significant VF loss in the nerve fiber bundle region extending across contiguously abnormal test points from the blind spot to at least 1 point outside of 15° adjacent to the nasal meridian.
High myopia-related detects	Enlarged blind spot	At least 2 abnormal test points with $P < 0.05$ contiguous with the blind spot and at least 1 worse than $P < 0.01$ in the pattern deviation plot
	Vertical step	Limited VE loss that respects the vertical meridian. Includes at least 2 abnormal test points located at or outside of 15° along the vertical meridian.
	Partial peripheral rim	General continuous field loss located outside of 15° showing some curved shape but not in all quadrants.
	Non-specific defect	A VF defect that does not belong to another detect type or classification.
Combined detects	Nasal step with enlarged blind spot	Nasal step paired with enlarged blind spot in the field.

VF: visual field

*A reproducible (in at least 2 consecutive reliable tests) reduction in sensitivity at a cluster of 2 or more contiguous test points with $P < 0.01$ loss or more or a cluster of 3 or more contiguous test points with $P < 0.05$ loss or more in the pattern deviation plot in the superior or interior arcuate areas, or a 10-dB difference across the nasal horizontal midline at a cluster of 2 or more adjacent test points in the total deviation plot.
**Point with $P < 0.05$ loss or more in the pattern deviation plot.
Reproduced from Lin F. *et al.*[34]

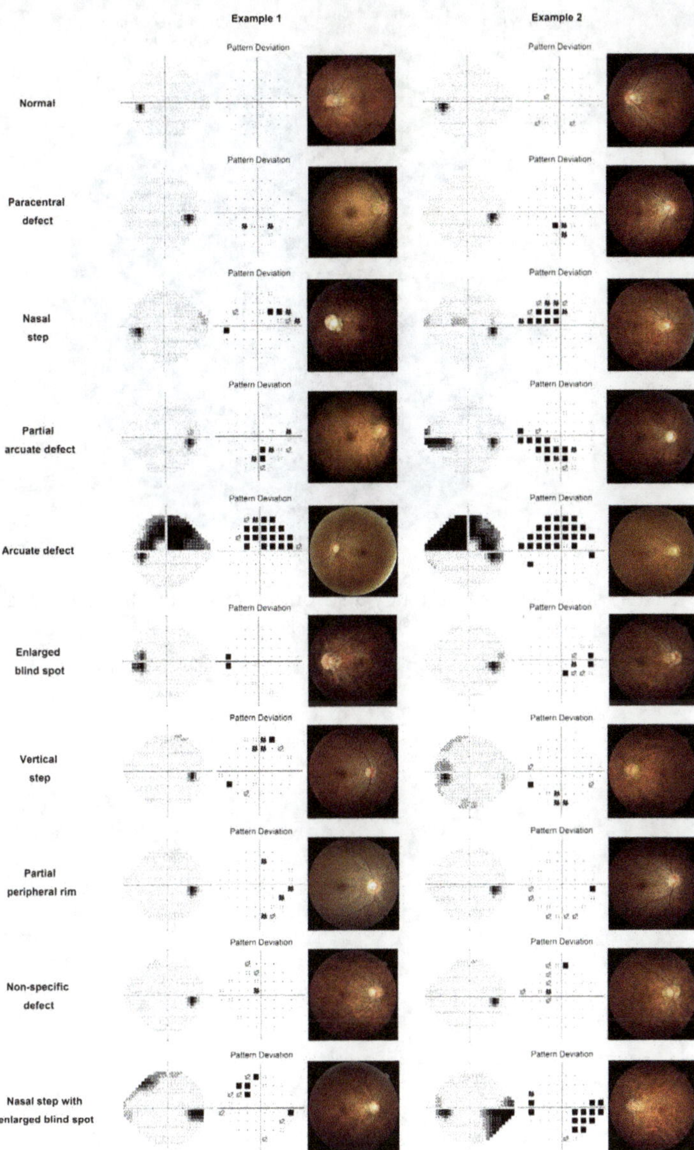

Fig. 1-11. Examples of the visual field abnormality classification with corresponding fundus photographs. Reproduced from Lin *et al.*[34]

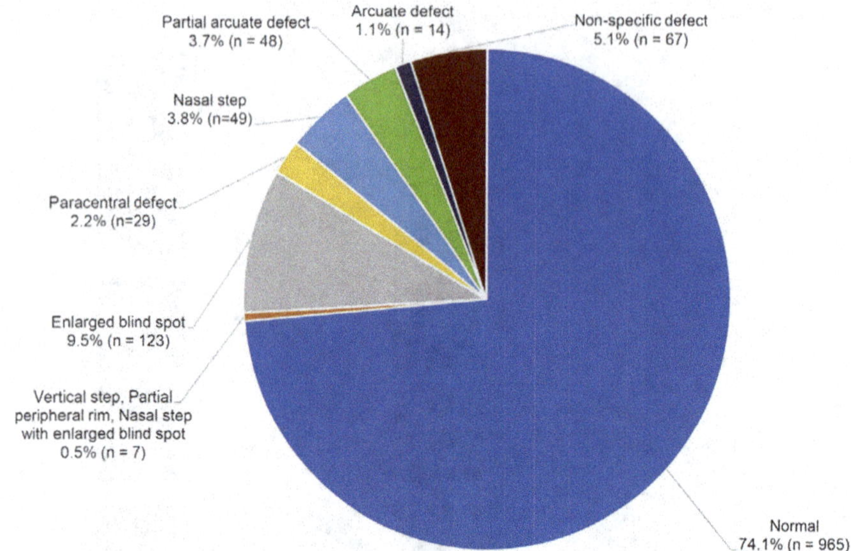

Fig. 1-12. Pie chart showing the frequency distribution of each visual field type in highly myopic eyes. Reproduced from Lin *et al.*[34]

References

1. Keltner JL, Johnson CA, Cello KE, Edwards MA, Bandermann SE, Kass MA, Gordon MO; Ocular Hypertension Treatment Study Group. Classification of visual field abnormalities in the ocular hypertension treatment study. Arch Ophthalmol. 2003 May;121(5):643-50. https://doi.org/10.1001/archopht.121.5.643

2. Balcer LJ, Prasad S. Abnormalities of the Optic Nerve and Retina. Available from: https://clinicalgate.com/abnormalities-of-the-optic-nerve-and-retina/

3. Bizios D, Heijl A, Bengtsson B. Integration and fusion of standard automated perimetry and optical coherence tomography data for improved automated glaucoma diagnostics. BMC Ophthalmol. 2011;11:20. https://doi.org/10.1186/1471-2415-11-20

4. Hood DC. Improving our understanding, and detection, of glaucomatous damage: An approach based upon optical coherence tomography (OCT). Prog Retin Eye Res. 2017 Mar;57:46-75. https://doi.org/10.1016/j.preteyeres.2017.01.002

5. Hood DC, Raza AS, de Moraes CG, Johnson CA, Liebmann JM, Ritch R. The nature of macular damage in glaucoma as revealed by averaging optical coherence tomography data. Transl Vis Sci Technol. 2012;1(1):3. https://doi.org/10.1167/tvst.1.1.3

6. Hood DC, Raza AS, de Moraes CG, Liebmann JM, Ritch R. Glaucomatous damage of the macula. Prog Retin Eye Res. 2013;32:1-21. https://doi.org/10.1016/j.preteyeres.2012.08.003

7. Kolker AE. Visual prognosis in advanced glaucoma: a comparison of medical and surgical therapy for retention of vision in 101 eyes with advanced glaucoma. Trans Am Ophthalmol Soc. 1977;75:539-55.

8. Kim JM, Kyung H, Shim SH, Azarbod P, Caprioli J. Location of initial visual field defects in glaucoma and their modes of deterioration. Invest Ophthalmol Vis Sci. 2015 Dec;56(13):7956-62. https://doi.org/10.1167/iovs.15-17297

9. Aulhorn E, Harms H. Early visual field defects in glaucoma. Published 1 July 1967.

10. Drance SM. The early field defects in glaucoma. Invest Ophthalmol. 1969 Feb;8(1):84-91. PMID: 5763849.

11. Heijl A, Lundqvist L. The frequency distribution of earliest glaucomatous visual field defects documented by automatic perimetry. Acta Ophthalmol (Copenh). 1984 Aug;62(4):658-64. https://doi.org/10.1111/j.1755-3768.1984.tb03979.x

12. Hood DC, Raza AS, de Moraes CG, et al. Initial arcuate defects within the central 10 degrees in glaucoma. Invest Ophthalmol Vis Sci. 2011;52:940-6. https://doi.org/10.1167/iovs.10-5803

13. Langerhorst C, Carenini L, Bakker D, et al. Measurements for description of very early glaucomatous field defects. Perimetry Update 1996/1997. New York, NY: Kugler Publications; 1997:67-73.

14. Schiefer U, Papageorgiou E, Sample PA, Pascual JP, Selig B, Krapp E, Paetzold J. Spatial pattern of glaucomatous visual field loss obtained with regionally condensed stimulus arrangements. Invest Ophthalmol Vis Sci. 2010 Nov;51(11):5685-9. https://doi.org/10.1167/iovs.09-5067

15. Caprioli J, Spaeth GL. Comparison of visual field defects in the low-tension glaucomas with those in the high-tension glaucomas. Am J Ophthalmol. 1984;97:730-7. https://doi.org/10.1016/0002-9394(84)90505-1

16. McKean-Cowdin R, Wang Y, Wu J, Azen SP, Varma R; Los Angeles Latino Eye Study Group. Impact of visual field loss on health-related quality of life in glaucoma: the Los Angeles Latino Eye Study. Ophthalmology. 2008;115:941-8. https://doi.org/10.1016/j.ophtha.2007.08.037

17. Yanagisawa M, Kato S, Kobayashi M, Watanabe M, Ochiai M. Relationship between vision-related quality of life and different types of existing visual fields in Japanese patients. Int Ophthalmol. 2012;32:523-9. https://doi.org/10.1007/s10792-012-9581-x

18. Fujita K, Yasuda N, Oda K, Yuzawa M. Reading performance in patients with central visual field disturbance due to glaucoma [in Japanese]. Nippon Ganka Gakkai Zasshi. 2006;110:914-8.

19. Coexkelbergh TR, Brouwer WH, Cornelissen FW, et al. The effect of visual field defects on driving performance: a driving simulator study. Arch Ophthalmol. 2002;120:1509-16. https://doi.org/10.1001/archopht.120.11.1509

20. Park SC, De Moraes CG, Teng CC, Tello C, Liebmann JM, Ritch R. Initial parafoveal versus peripheral scotomas in glaucoma: risk factors and visual field characteristics. Ophthalmology. 2011 Sep;118(9):1782-9. https://doi.org/10.1016/j.ophtha.2011.02.013

21. Jung KI, Park HY, Park CK. Characteristics of optic disc morphology in glaucoma patients with parafoveal scotoma compared to peripheral scotoma. Invest Ophthalmol Vis Sci. 2012 Jul 20;53(8):4813-20. https://doi.org/10.1167/iovs.12-9908

22. Kosior-Jarecka E, Wróbel-Dudzińska D, Łukasik U, Żarnowski T. Zmiany w polu widzenia w przebiegu jaskry z normalnym ciśnieniem i ich związek z obecnością czynników ryzyka [Visual field changes in normal pressure glaucoma and their association with risk factors]. Klin Oczna. 2016;118(3):208-13. Polish. PMID: 30088385.

23. Hitchings RA, Anderton SA. A comparative study of visual field defects seen in patients with low-tension glaucoma and chronic simple glaucoma. Br J Ophthalmol. 1983 Dec;67(12):818-21. https://doi.org/10.1136/bjo.67.12.818

24. Weinreb RN, Aung T, Medeiros FA. The pathophysiology and treatment of glaucoma: a review. JAMA. 2014;311(18):1901-11.https://doi.org/10.1001/jama.2014.3192

25. Broadway DC, Nicolela MT, Drance SM. Optic disk appearances in primary open-angle glaucoma. Surv Ophthalmol. 1999;43 Suppl 1.https://doi.org/10.1016/S0039-6257(99)00007-7

26. Nicolela MT, Drance SM. Various glaucomatous optic nerve appearances: clinical correlations. Ophthalmology. 1996;103(4):640-9. https://doi.org/10.1016/S0161-6420(96)30513-7

27. Reis AS, Artes PH, Belliveau AC, et al. Rates of change in the visual field and optic disc in patients with distinct patterns of glaucomatous optic disc damage. Ophthalmology. 2012;119(2):294-303. https://doi.org/10.1016/j.ophtha.2011.07.044

28. Nicolela MT, McCormick TA, Drance SM, Ferrier SN, LeBlanc RP, Chauhan BC. Visual field and optic disc progression in patients with different types of optic disc damage: a longitudinal prospective study. Ophthalmology. 2003;110(11):2178-84. https://doi.org/10.1016/S0161-6420(03)00801-7

29. Curcio CA, Allen KA. Topography of ganglion cells in human retina. J Comp Neurol. 1990;300(1):5-25. https://doi.org/10.1002/cne.903000103

30. Pan CW, Cheung CY, Aung T, et al. Differential associations of myopia with major age-related eye diseases: the Singapore Indian Eye Study. Ophthalmology. 2013;120:284-291. https://doi.org/10.1016/j.ophtha.2012.07.065

31. Marcus MW, de Vries MM, Junoy Montolio FG, Jansonius NM. Myopia as a risk factor for open-angle glaucoma: a systematic review and meta-analysis. Ophthalmology. 2011;118:1989-1994.e1982. https://doi.org/10.1016/j.ophtha.2011.03.012

32. Jonas JB, Weber P, Nagaoka N, Ohno-Matsui K. Glaucoma in high myopia and parapapillary delta zone. PLoS One. 2017;12: e0175120. https://doi.org/10.1371/journal.pone.0175120

33. Lanca C, Sun CH, Chong R, et al. Visual field defects and myopic macular degeneration in Singapore adults with high myopia. Br J Ophthalmol. 2022;106:1423-1428. https://doi.org/10.1136/bjophthalmol-2020-318674

34. Lin F, Chen S, Song Y, et al. Classification of Visual Field Abnormalities in Highly Myopic Eyes without Pathologic Change. Ophthalmology. 2022 Jul;129(7):803-812. https://doi.org/10.1016/j.ophtha.2022.03.001

35. Aref AA, Budenz DL. Detecting visual field progression. Ophthalmology. 2017;124:S51-S56. https://doi.org/10.1016/j.ophtha.2017.05.010

36. Kapoor R, Yuksel-Elgin C, Patel V, et al. Detecting common eye diseases using the first teleophthalmology globechek kiosk in the United States: a pilot study. Asia Pac J Ophthalmol (Phila). 2020;9:315-325. https://doi.org/10.1097/APO.0000000000000295

37. Heijl A, Leske MC, Bengtsson B, et al. Reduction of intraocular pressure and glaucoma progression: results from the Early Manifest Glaucoma Trial. Arch Ophthalmol. 2002;120: 1268-1279. https://doi.org/10.1001/archopht.120.10.1268

38. Kass MA, Heuer DK, Higginbotham EJ, et al. The Ocular Hypertension Treatment Study: a randomized trial determines that topical ocular hypotensive medication delays or

prevents the onset of primary open-angle glaucoma. Arch Ophthalmol. 2002;120:701-713. discussion 829-830. https://doi.org/10.1001/archopht.120.6.701

39. Garway-Heath DF, Crabb DP, Bunce C, et al. Latanoprost for open-angle glaucoma (UKGTS): a randomised, multicentre, placebo-controlled trial. Lancet. 2015;385:1295-1304. https://doi.org/10.1016/S0140-6736(14)62111-5

Chapter 2

Understanding central visual field defects in early glaucoma

This chapter provides an understanding of CVFDs in the central 10° of the VF in early glaucoma on 24-2 VF. Early glaucoma is defined here as MD better than -6 dB. This damage can also be expressed as glaucomatous damage of the macula in the early stage of glaucoma,[1,2] based on structural changes in the central 8°–10°.

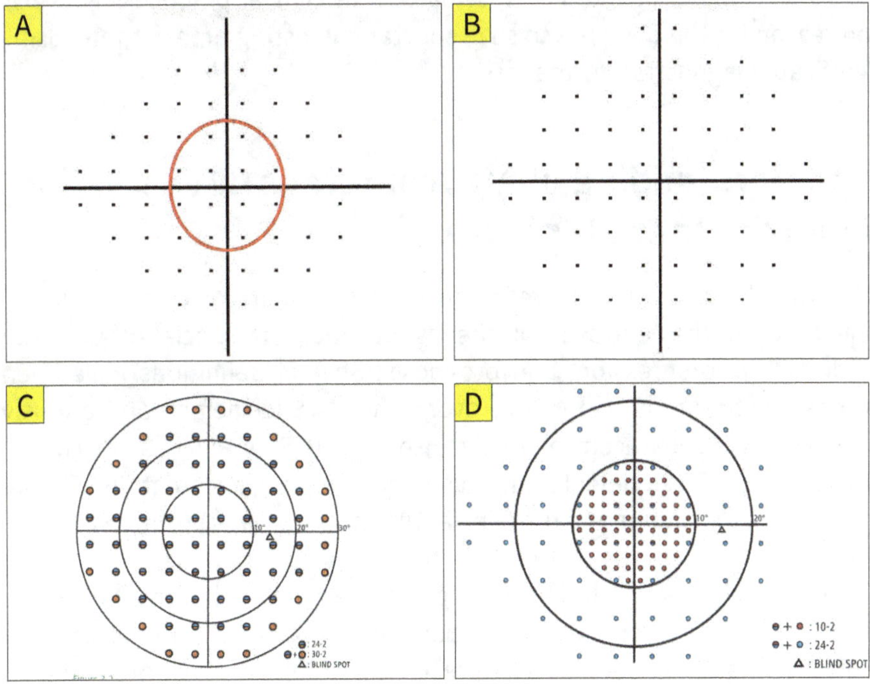

Fig. 2-1. (A) The test points in 24-2 VF and central 12 points within central 10° (outlined in red). **(B)** The 68 points in a 10-2 test pattern, representing test point locations in the central 10°. **(C)** Comparison of the 30-2 and 24-2 test point locations. Test points are set 6° apart. Reproduced from Heijl *et al.*[3] **(D)** Comparison between the 24-2 and 10-2 test patterns. Reproduced from Heijl *et al.*[3]

1. Standard test pattern and test point locations in 24-2 VF test

A 24-2 Size III White SITA Standard Threshold Test usually is the best choice for a perimetric test for glaucoma patients. Hence, our discussion on CVFD is based on the 24-2 VF test pattern. For a better understanding, we describe here the test point locations in 30-2 and 24-2 test grids (Fig. 2-1). The HFA 30-2 pattern measures visual sensitivity at 76 locations within 30° of fixation (Fig. 2-1C). The 24-2 test pattern consists of 54 test points which are spaced 6° apart(Fig. 2-1A). Of 54 test locations, 52 are within the central 24° plus 2 nasal locations near 30°. The innermost 12 test locations lie within the central 10° around fixation. Over time, the 24-2 test pattern has substituted the 76 test points of the 30-2 test pattern in clinical practice (Fig. 2-1C). The reason for this switch is to save substantial testing time without losing significant diagnostic information.

2. Understanding of glaucomatous CFVDs in the light of extant literature

There has been a surge of research interest in initial glaucomatous VF defects within the central 10° in the last decade, with special reference to its detection, progression, and prognosis. Several definitions have been proposed in the literature for CVFD over the years. Such defects are variously known as CVFDs, paracentral defects, isolated IPFS, or PFS (also discussed in Chapter 1). These defects have also been called glaucomatous arcuate defects, largely confined to the central 10° on achromatic perimetry.

Research has shown that in some glaucoma patients in the early stages of the disease, glaucomatous macular defects can be present and the central VF may be affected, even as an initial VF defect.[4-7] Previous research demonstrated that in eyes with open-angle glaucoma, the earliest changes detected with the help of static perimetry were paracentral scotomas in the Bjerrum area separated from the blind spot, merging into an arcuate scotoma joining the blind spot.[8]

In a study designed explicitly to evaluate initial glaucomatous defects, nearly 3000 eyes with ocular hypertension, with or without established glaucoma in the fellow eye, were followed with automatic perimetry for several years. Forty-five eyes showed a documented change from repeated normal VFs to reproducible glaucomatous VF loss.[9] There were several abnormal points at the central 5°, especially nasally and in the superior hemifield. Nasal VF damage is often one of the earliest sites of glaucomatous functional loss. Another study reported that over 50% of eyes with mild to moderate glaucoma had defects within the central ± 3°.[10]

3. Types and patterns of defects considered glaucomatous CVFDs on 24-2 VF

The VF status of these eyes is early glaucomatous defects, (with MD ≤ -6dB) as per classification based on MD staging of 24-2 VF tests (Figs. 2-2, 2-3).

3.1. Isolated IPFS

IPFS is defined as a glaucomatous VF defect in 1 hemifield with 3 adjacent points with $P < 5\%$ within the central 10° of fixation, with at least 1 point at $P < 1\%$ lying at the innermost paracentral points and no VF abnormality outside the central 10° degrees (Figs. 2-2, 2-3A).[11]

3.2. PFS within the central 10°

Some research divided the initial VF defects on the PD plot of the 24-2 VF test pattern into 2 groups (Fig. 2-2B): paracentral defect, where the points are lying from 0° to 10°, and nasal defect for points beyond 20° (see Chapter 1).[12]

3.3. Abnormal single-point defect depressed $P < 1\%$ within the central-most 4 points

An abnormal single-point defect ($P < 1\%$) present on 3 consecutive tests on 24-2VF within the central 5°, but not part of a cluster, may be considered a CVFD (Fig. 2-3B).[13] It should be considered that test-retest variability is typically the lowest at the most central points of the VF than at peripheral points.[14] Previous studies have also reported cases where a single abnormal point defect within the 4 innermost points of the 24-2 VF turned out to be an arcuate-like PFS on a 10-2 VF test.[15]

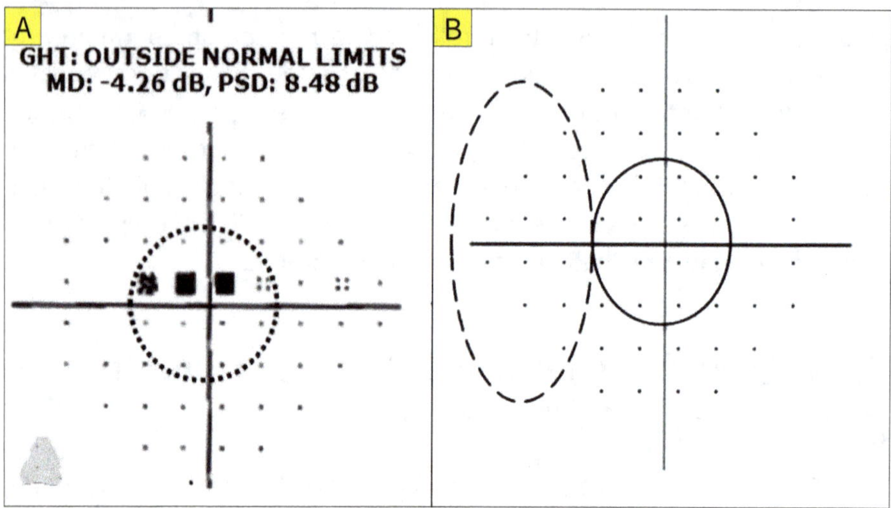

Fig. 2-2. (A) Examples of an isolated IPFS limited to 1 hemifield within the dashed circle. Reproduced from Park *et al.*[11] **(B)** PFS and PNS. The PFS group includes abnormal points within 12 points of a central 10° radius (circle). The PNS group has abnormal points within 12 nasal peripheral points (dashed line) in 1 hemifield. Reproduced from Jung *et al.*[12]

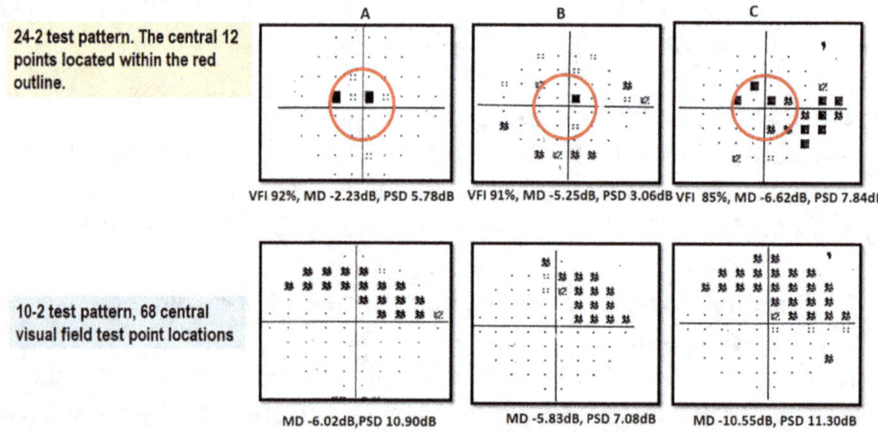

Fig. 2-3. Different types and patterns of CVFDs on 24-2 VF and corresponding 10-2 VF defects related to initial defects. The MD and particularly the PSD value in the 10-2 test results are worse in each case than the MD and PSD of the initial 24-2 test results. Reproduced from Chakravarti *et al.*[13]

3.4. Abnormal central point defect in a cluster within the central 10° where the cluster extends beyond the central 10°

Abnormal points within a cluster (3 contiguous points: 5%, 5%, 1%) in the central 10°, but that cluster extending beyond the central 10° either on the TD or PD plot within a hemifield on 24-2 VF can be considered CVFDs, as shown in Figure 2-3C.[16] However, such defects are not considered as CVFD by some researchers.[2]

3.5. Abnormal VF points within the central 12 points

Abnormal 24-2 VF points depressed either < 5%, < 2%, < 1%, or < 0.5% from the normal database on PD plot are considered CVFD.[17]

Table 2-1. Definition of CVFDs on a 24-2 VF (MD ≤ 6 dB) based on the following criteria

Definition based on point or cluster criteria	Defined either by the presence of abnormal 24-2 VF points or cluster formed by the abnormal points in the central 10°.
Definition based on abnormalities in probability plot criteria	Defined based on abnormalities either on the PD probability plot, the TD plot, or both.
Definition based on abnormal points' probability value	The definition included abnormal 24-2 VF point probability values: < 0.5%, < 1%, < 2%, < 5%.
Definition based on structural and functional agreement	Glaucomatous macular damage is based on the topographic agreement between the VF results and RGC + IPL probability plots.

4. Evolving definitions of CVFDs on 24-2 VF (MD ≤ -6 dB) from the published literature

4.1. Hood *et al.*

Several definitions have been suggested over the years for CVFDs based on the criteria listed in Table 2-1. Listed below are 5 definitions associated with the concept of CVFD on 24-2 VF based on the criteria described in Table 2-1. Included abnormal points or clusters within central 10° (central 12 points) and excluded those with defects outside the central 10° on the 24-2 test.[2] They included included eyes with an arcuate defect on 10-2 VF if the 24-2 test was normal outside the central 10°. Fig. 2-4 shows the region of the 24-2

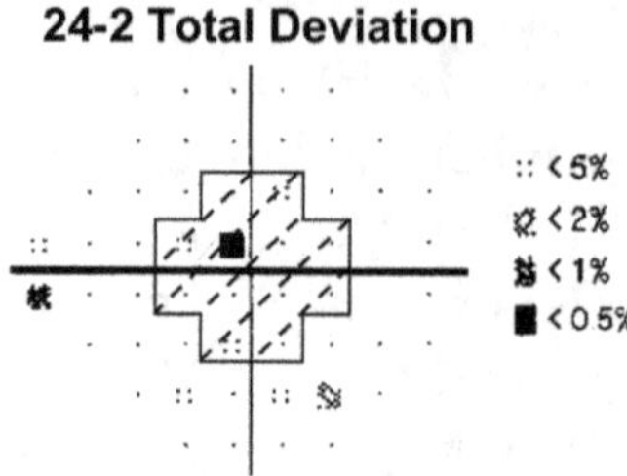

Fig. 2-4. The 24-2 test pattern shows the region (dashed diagonal lines) represented by the 10-2 test pattern. Reproduced from Hood *et al.*[2]

test pattern represented by the 10-2 test pattern. They included structural analysis, plots of RNFL thickness of the macula.

4.2. Garg *et al.*

Any of the 12 central-most points with TD values at $P < 0.5\%$ on 2 consecutive examinations.[18]

4.3. Grilo *et al.*

Cluster criteria: Three neighboring points at 5%, 5%, and 1% or 5%, 2%, and 2% probability or worse within a hemifield on TD or PD plots, with only 1 point allowed on the edge of the 24-2. Macular points within ± 10°: 1 point at 1% or 2 points at 2% within a hemifield on TD or PD.[19]

4.4. Roberti *et al.*

Criteria for a CVFD within the central 10° VF area of the HFA 24-2 test was defined with the presence of a cluster of 3 significantly depressed contiguous points with $P < 5\%$ in at least 2 test locations, and $P < 2\%$ in at least 1 test location within the central 12 test point area.[20]

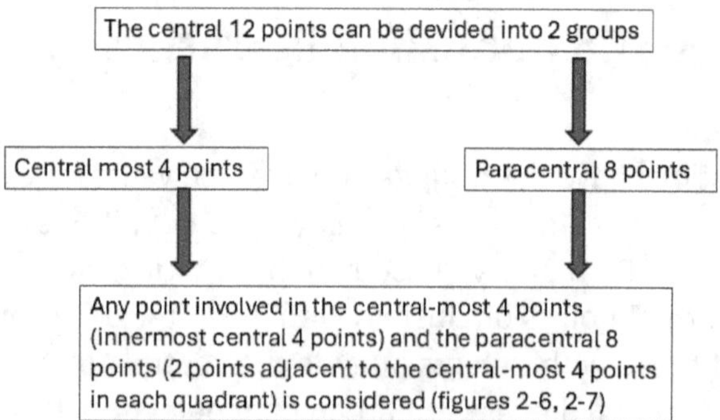

Fig. 2-5. Defining central and paracentral points within the central 12 points.

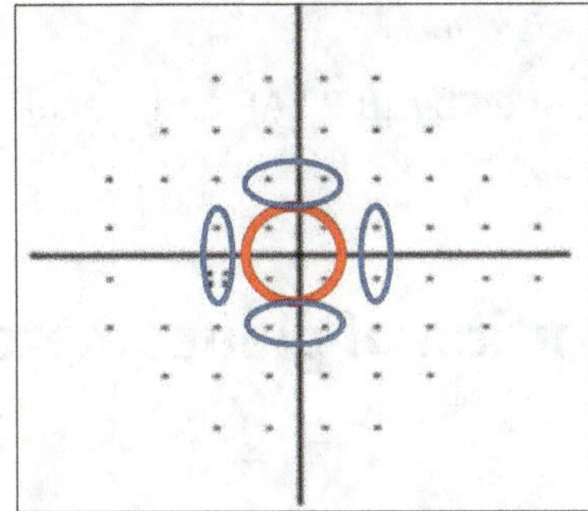

Fig. 2-6. Central and paracentral points within the central 10°. The innermost central 4 points are encircled with red color and the paracentral 8 points (2 points adjacent to the central-most 4 points in each quadrant) are encircled with blue color.

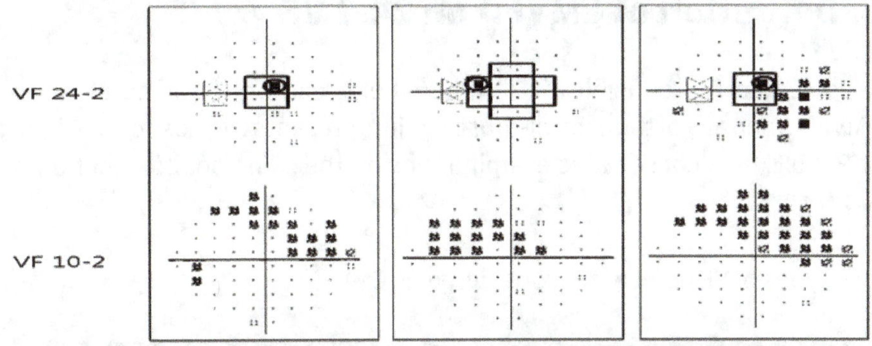

Fig. 2-7. Representative cases with abnormal VF points (central and paracentral) depressed < 0.5% from the normative database within the central 12 points on the HFA 24-2 VF test. **(Left)** A case with an abnormal 24-2 VF point depressed < 0.5% (black box) within the central 4 points showing a PFS on the 10-2 VF test. **(Middle)** A case with an abnormal VF point depressed < 0.5% (black box) within the paracentral 8 points showing a PFS on the 10-2 VF test. **(Right)** A case with an inferior arcuate VF defect with an additional superior abnormal point depressed < 0.5% **(black box)** within the superior innermost central 4 points. This case has a superior PFS on the 10-2 VF test that was not evident on the 24-2 VF test. Reproduced from Park *et al.*[21]

4.5. De Moraes *et al.*

Macular damage was defined by 10-2 SAP and macular SD-OCT evidence of RGC + IPL probability maps.[1]

5. A recent definition of glaucomatous CVFD on 24-2 VF

CVFD is defined as abnormal VF points depressed < 1% or < 0.5% from the normal database within the central 12 points (in the central 10°) on TD or PD probability plots on a 24-2 VF test (Figs. 2-5, 2-6, 2-7).[15]

6. Definition of CMVFD on 24-2 VF

Reliable and reproducible 24-2 VF hemifields can be classified as having CMVFD when any of the central-most 4 points presents with loss of sensitivity at $P < 1\%$, on 3 consecutive examinations on the same points either on TD or PD plots.[13]

Two types of VF defects are considered as CMVFD:

1. Type 1 involves eyes with an isolated IPFS (Figs. 2-2A, 2-3A). Further, an abnormal single-point defect with $P < 1\%$ within the central-most 4 points but not being a part of a cluster, is also considered as CMVFD (Fig. 2-3B).

2. Type 2 involves a combined defect where an IPFS is merged with a peripheral defect. Figure 2-8 illustrates all the types of CMVFDs on 24-2 VF.[13]

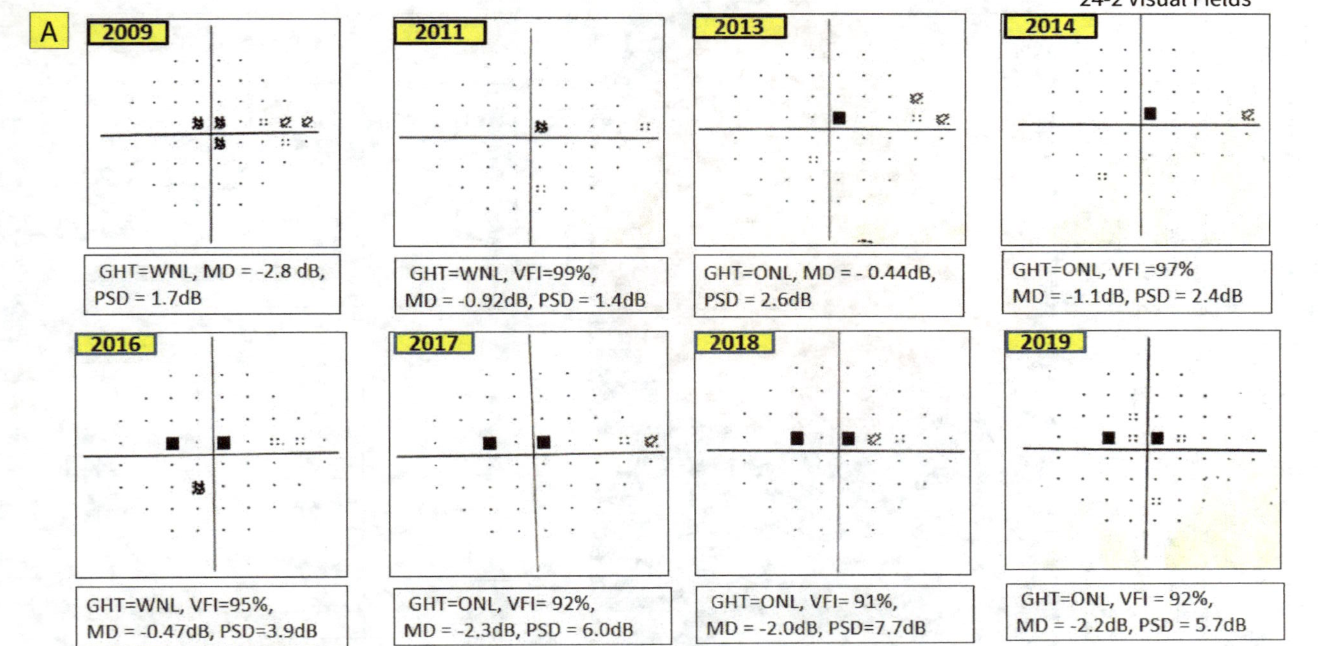

Fig. 2-8. This figure relates to how an initial central-most VF defect transformed into an arcuate defect. **(A)** This case is of a 40-year-old male with NTG who has been followed for over 14 years. His untreated IOP was 18–19 mmHg bilaterally and his earliest VF defect (2009) was only a central-most VF defect in his left eye. On 3 consecutive examinations from 2011 to 2014, his left eye showed a single abnormal point, $P < 0.5\%$, within the central 5° in the superior nasal hemifield on the PD probability plot. GHT failed to recognize any abnormality in the first 2 VFs with central-most VF defects and interpreted those VFs as Within Normal Limits (2009, 2011). The standard metrics (MD, PSD, VFI) underrated early glaucomatous damage from 2009 to 2016. He presented with an initial PFS-like defect in 2018 in the superior hemifield within the central 10° on 24-2 VF.

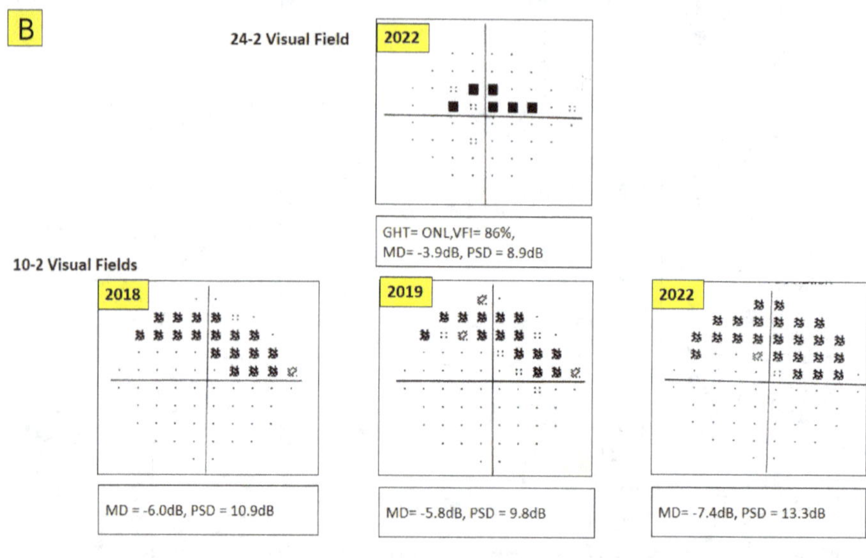

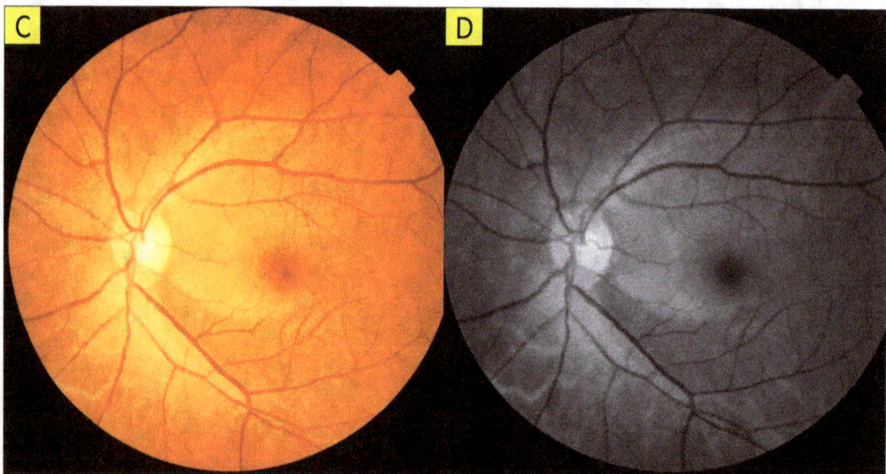

Fig. 2-8. Continued. **(B)** The progression of VF loss in the same eye was detected in 2022. In 2022, his VFI (86%) decreased by 14% but the severity of visual loss was not reflected in the MD value (-3.9 dB). However, the PSD was high, 8.9 dB. When tested with a 10-2 VF test, the same eye showed an arcuate scotoma from 2018 to 2022 and revealed the severity of the CVFD in this eye. The MD and PSD values of the 10-2 VF test were much worse than the initial 24-2 VF results. Hence, 10-2 VF testing is critical for a proper understanding of the significance of this type of defect. **(C)** Fundus photograph (2018) of the patient's left eye showing a localized, wedge-shaped RNFL defect in the inferior temporal quadrant. **(D)** Red-free fundus photograph of the left eye shows RNFL wedge defect inferotemporal to disc. The localised RNFL defects occur most often in NTG, followed by POAG.

7. The importance of a 10-2 VF test in patients with a high risk of CVFDs

The 10-2 VF test is considered the most beneficial to evaluate early glaucoma CVFDs in the cases described in Figures 2-7 and 2-8. Evidence suggests that a testing algorithm such as the 10-2 VF test with closely spaced grids of 68 points spaced 2° apart, is more effective and demonstrates superior performance compared with the 24-2 VF test for detecting CVFDs and/or glaucomatous macular damage in the central 10° in early glaucoma (see Chapter 5).[22]

8. Central VF damage affects health-related QoL

Glaucoma affects both central and mid-peripheral vision. Patients with VF damage in the central 10° would likely have greater disability in visual function than those with preserved central VF. Therefore, using only 24-2 and/or 30-2 VF assessments of visual function may underestimate the extent, location, and implication of glaucomatous VF loss.

A broad range of activities such as reading, driving, and walking outside the home are significantly impaired by glaucoma.[23-27] Glaucoma impacts health-related QoL in multiple ways, including driving,[28] walking and falls,[29] and reading involving central and near vision.[30] Moreover, central vision — which correlates with macular function— is important when performing activities of daily life. Given the high density of RGCs in the macula and their overwhelming representation in the visual cortex, it is expected that damage to the macula can substantially affect health-related QoL.

9. Glaucomatous central VF damage and vision-related QoL

The US National Eye Institute Visual Function Questionnaire (NEI VFQ-25) evaluates vision-related QOL and was designed to assess the extent of self-reported vision that is relevant for patients with chronic eye diseases. It consists of 25 questions representing 11 subscales plus an additional single-item general health-rating question. The subscales are general vision, near and distance vision activities, ocular pain, vision-related social function, vision-related role function, vision-related mental health, vision-related dependency, driving difficulties, color vision, and peripheral vision. Each subscale consists of 1 to 4 items.

Recent research investigated and compared the association between NEI VFQ-25 scores and VF status as measured by the 10-2 and 24-2 VF tests.[31] This cross-sectional cohort study included 113 glaucoma patients with the entire range of 24-2 VF damage who completed the NEI VFQ-25. Interviewers administered the NEI VFQ-25 survey on the same day that the VF tests were performed. The findings of this study suggest that 10-2 VF tests show a stronger association with NEI VFQ-25 scores than do 24-2 VF tests. Patients with disproportionately poor NEI VFQ-25 scores, despite relatively good binocular 24-2 VF results may have central VF damage on 10-2 VF testing.

Another study demonstrated that vision-specific QOL begins to decline with mild VF loss and continues to decline with increasing severity of VF loss.[32] The largest impact of VF loss on health-related QOL was seen in patients with any central VF loss. Health-related QOL is diminished even in persons with relatively mild VF loss based on MD scores. Large effects were most frequently found for participants with central or central and peripheral VF loss, whereas moderate to large effects were found for 5 of 12 NEI-VFQ subscales and the composite score for participants with bilateral peripheral VF loss. The lower health-related QOL scores for glaucoma participants with any central VF loss fit with the disease course progressing from peripheral VF loss in the early stages of the disease to central and peripheral VF loss in the more advanced stages of the disease.

References

1. De Moraes CG, Sun A, Jarukasetphon R, et al. Association of macular visual field measurements with glaucoma staging systems. JAMA Ophthalmol. 2019 Feb;137(2):139-145. https://doi.org/10.1001/jamaophthalmol.2018.5398

2. Hood DC, Raza AS, de Moraes CG, Odel JG, Greenstein VC, Liebmann JM, Ritch R. Initial arcuate defects within the central 10 degrees in glaucoma. Invest Ophthalmol Vis Sci. 2011 Feb 16;52(2):940-6. https://doi.org/10.1167/iovs.10-5803

3. Heijl A, Vincent Patella VM, Bengtsson B. The Field Analyzer Primer: Excellent Perimetry, 5th Edition. Carl Zeiss Meditec; 2021.

4. Drance SM. The early field defects in glaucoma. Invest Ophthalmol. 1969;8(1):84-91.

5. Hood DC, Raza AS, de Moraes CG, et al. Initial arcuate defects within the central 10 degrees in glaucoma. Invest Ophthalmol Vis Sci. 2011;52:940-946. https://doi.org/10.1167/iovs.10-5803

6. Hood DC, Raza AS, de Moraes CG, et al. Glaucomatous damage of the macula. Prog Retin Eye Res. 2013;32:1-21. https://doi.org/10.1016/j.preteyeres.2012.08.003

7. Langerhorst C, Carenini L, Bakker D, et al. Measurements for description of very early glaucomatous field defects. Perimetry Update 1996/1997. New York, NY: Kugler; 1997:67-73.

8. Kosaki H. The earliest visual field defect (IIa stage) in glaucoma by kinetic perimetry. In: Greve EL, editor. Third International Visual Field Symposium Tokyo, May 3-6, 1978. Documenta Ophthalmologica Proceedings Series, vol 19. Springer, Dordrecht; 1979. https://doi.org/10.1007/978-94-009-9611-3_28

9. Heijl A, Lundqvist L. The frequency distribution of earliest glaucomatous visual field defects documented by automatic perimetry. Acta Ophthalmol (Copenh). 1984;62(4):658-664. https://doi.org/10.1111/j.1755-3768.1984.tb03979.x

10. Schiefer U, Papageorgiou E, Sample PA, et al. Spatial pattern of glaucomatous visual field loss obtained with regionally condensed stimulus arrangements. Invest Ophthalmol Vis Sci. 2010;51(11):5685-5689. https://doi.org/10.1167/iovs.09-5067

11. Park SC, De Moraes CG, Teng CC, Tello C, Liebmann JM, Ritch R. Initial parafoveal versus peripheral scotomas in glaucoma: risk factors and visual field characteristics. Ophthalmology. 2011;118:1782-1789. https://doi.org/10.1016/j.ophtha.2011.02.013

12. Jung KI, Park HY, Park CK. Characteristics of optic disc morphology in glaucoma patients with parafoveal scotoma compared to peripheral scotoma. Invest Ophthalmol Vis Sci. 2012 Jul 20;53(8):4813-20. https://doi.org/10.1167/iovs.12-9908

13. Chakravarti T, Moghimi S, De Moraes CG, Weinreb RN. Central-most visual field defects in early glaucoma. J Glaucoma. 2021 Mar 1;30(3). https://doi.org/10.1097/IJG.0000000000001747

14. Heijl A, Leske MC, Bengtsson B, et al. Test-retest variability in glaucomatous visual fields. Am J Ophthalmol. 1989;108:130-135. https://doi.org/10.1016/0002-9394(89)90006-8

15. Park HY, Hwang BE, Shin HY, Park CK. Clinical clues to predict the presence of parafoveal scotoma on Humphrey 10-2 visual field using a Humphrey 24-2 visual field. Am J Ophthalmol. 2016;161:150-159. https://doi.org/10.1016/j.ajo.2015.10.007

16. Chakravarti T, Moghimi S, Weinreb RN. Prediction of central visual field severity in glaucoma. J Glaucoma. 2022 Jun;31(6):430-437. https://doi.org/10.1097/IJG.0000000000002031

17. Park HY, Hwang BE, Shin HY, Park CK. Clinical clues to predict the presence of parafoveal scotoma on Humphrey 10-2 visual field using a Humphrey 24-2 visual field. Am J Ophthalmol. 2016;161:150-159. https://doi.org/10.1016/j.ajo.2015.10.007

18. Garg A, De Moraes CG, Cioffi GA, Girkin CA, Medeiros FA, Weinreb RN, Zangwill LM, Liebmann JM. Baseline 24-2 central visual field damage is predictive of global progressive field loss. Am J Ophthalmol. 2018 Mar;187:92-98. https://doi.org/10.1016/j.ajo.2018.01.001

19. Grillo LM, Wang DL, Ramachandran R, Ehrlich AC, De Moraes CG, Ritch R, Hood DC. The 24-2 visual field test misses central macular damage confirmed by the 10-2 visual field test and optical coherence tomography. Transl Vis Sci Technol. 2016 Apr 14;5(2):15. https://doi.org/10.1167/tvst.5.2.15

20. Roberti G, Manni G, Riva I, Holló G, Quaranta L, Agnifili L, Figus M, Giammaria S, Rastelli D, Oddone F. Detection of central visual field defects in early glaucomatous eyes: comparison of Humphrey and Octopus perimetry. PLoS One. 2017 Oct 27;12(10) https://doi.org/10.1371/journal.pone.0186793

21. Park HY, Hwang BE, Shin HY, Park CK. Clinical clues to predict the presence of parafoveal scotoma on Humphrey 10-2 visual field using a Humphrey 24-2 visual field. Am J Ophthalmol. 2016 Jan;161:150-9. https://doi.org/10.1016/j.ajo.2015.10.007

22. Traynis I, De Moraes CG, Raza AS, Liebmann JM, Ritch R, Hood DC. Prevalence and nature of early glaucomatous defects in the central 10° of the visual field. JAMA Ophthalmol. 2014 Mar;132(3):291-7. https://doi.org/10.1001/jamaophthalmol.2013.7656

23. Parrish RK 2nd, Gedde SJ, Scott IU, et al. Visual function and quality of life among patients with glaucoma. Arch Ophthalmol. 1997;115:1447-1455. https://doi.org/10.1001/archopht.1997.01100160617016

24. Mills RP, Janz NK, Wren PA, Guire KE. Correlation of visual field with quality-of-life measures at diagnosis in the Collaborative Initial Glaucoma Treatment Study (CIGTS). J Glaucoma. 2001;10:192-198. https://doi.org/10.1097/00061198-200106000-00008

25. Ringsdorf L, McGwin G Jr, Owsley C. Visual field defects and vision-specific health-related quality of life in African Americans and whites with glaucoma. J Glaucoma. 2006;15:414-418. https://doi.org/10.1097/01.ijg.0000212252.72207.c2

26. Burr JM, Kilonzo M, Vale L, Ryan M. Developing a preference-based glaucoma utility index using a discrete choice experiment. Optom Vis Sci. 2007;84:797-808. https://doi.org/10.1097/OPX.0b013e3181339f30

27. Aspinall PA, Johnson ZK, Azuara-Blanco A, et al. Evaluation of quality of life and priorities of patients with glaucoma. Invest Ophthalmol Vis Sci. 2008;49:1907-1915. https://doi.org/10.1167/iovs.07-0559

28. Ramulu PY, West SK, Munoz B, et al. Driving cessation and driving limitation in glaucoma: the Salisbury Eye Evaluation Project. Ophthalmology. 2009;116:1846-1853. https://doi.org/10.1016/j.ophtha.2009.03.033

29. Baig S, Diniz-Filho A, Wu Z, et al. Association of fast visual field loss with risk of falling in patients with glaucoma. JAMA Ophthalmol. 2016. https://doi.org/10.1001/jamaophthalmol.2016.1659

30. Ramulu PY, West SK, Munoz B, et al. Glaucoma and reading speed: the Salisbury Eye Evaluation Project. Arch Ophthalmol. 2009;127:82-87. https://doi.org/10.1001/archophthalmol.2008.523

31. Blumberg DM, De Moraes CG, Prager AJ, Yu Q, Al-Aswad L, Cioffi GA, Liebmann JM, Hood DC. Association between undetected 10-2 visual field damage and vision-related quality of life in patients with glaucoma. JAMA Ophthalmol. 2017 Jul 1;135(7):742-747. https://doi.org/10.1001/jamaophthalmol.2017.1396

32. McKean-Cowdin R, Varma R, Wu J, Hays RD, Azen SP; Los Angeles Latino Eye Study Group. Severity of visual field loss and health-related quality of life. Am J Ophthalmol. 2007 Jun;143(6):1013-23. https://doi.org/10.1016/j.ajo.2007.02.022

Chapter 3

The structural aspect of detecting glaucomatous macular damage

This book focuses on an understanding of the functional aspects of CVFD, *i.e.*, glaucomatous macular damage. Consequently, our discussion is mostly restricted to the arena of perimetric tools for explaining CVFD. However, current research has extensively analyzed this defect, furnishing a plethora of information based on the structural damage of the macular area that underpins this research paradigm.[1] We have limited scope here to discuss all in detail. Hence, very briefly we touch on the structural aspect of detecting glaucomatous macular damage in early glaucoma.

The present chapter takes into account several studies that have evaluated the structure-function correlation of the 24-2 and 10-2 VF tests with RNFL and retinal ganglion cell layer plus inner plexiform layer (RGC + IPL). This chapter also presents a series of schematic models introduced to specify the relative vulnerability of optic disc regions to early glaucomatous damage.

1. Diagnostic ability of macular intraretinal layer thickness with cpRNFL thickness for detecting early, moderate, and advanced glaucoma

So far, a common protocol is to use the 24-2 VF test strategy in early-stage glaucoma and to use the 10-2 VF test strategy for later stages in cases where significant central VF damage is present. However, recent studies using OCT indicate that thinning within the macular ganglion cell complex often occurs early. Some investigators compared the diagnostic ability of macular intraretinal layer thickness with cpRNFL thickness, either when used individually or in combination with cpRNFL for detecting early, moderate, and advanced glaucoma.[2] They studied a total of 423 glaucoma participants and 423 age- and gender-matched normal participants. This study observed that combining macular measurements (GCL and GCL-IPL) and cpRNFL improved the diagnostic performance and differentation of early and moderate glaucoma (early glaucoma [AUC = 0.908; P = 0.002] and moderate glaucoma [AUC = 0.944; P = 0.031]), but not of advanced glaucoma (AUC = 0.991; P > 0.05). For the diagnosis of early and moderate glaucoma single-layer mGCL thickness is comparable to the traditional cpRNFL thickness. However, cpRNFL thickness remains the most efficient for diagnosing advanced glaucoma. They concluded that both macular and optic disc scans should be used to diagnose early glaucoma.

2. Structure-function correlation of 24-2 and 10-2 VF tests with mGCIPL thickness

While many studies have found that the 24-2 VF test underestimates macular damage, others have found the 24-2 VF test was comparable to the 10-2 in detecting macular damage in early glaucoma patients (MD ≤ -6 dB).

Park *et al.* compared 112 early glaucoma eyes with mGCIPL thinning on the deviation map of macular spectral-domain OCT (SD-OCT) with 35 normal controls.[3] They observed that FDT 10-2 had a better diagnostic capacity than FDT 24-2 for eyes with the average and minimum mGCIPL thicknesses depressed at the < 1% level and differentiating normal controls from glaucoma patients with macular damage. Comparing 10-2 and 24-2 tests with the same strategy, their findings indicated that FDT 10-2 was more sensitive than FDT 24-2 (P = 0.004), with better specificity (P = 0.010).

Hood *et al.* evaluated the agreement between structural (OCT) and functional (VF) glaucomatous damage with an automated method and deviation/probability maps and compared this method to a metric method.[4] They studied topographic agreement between VF and SD-OCT disc and mGCIPL scans among 53 eyes with definite early glaucoma and 45 healthy control eyes. The study defined abnormal OCT structure-abnormal VF function as 2 or more abnormal (< 5%) points on the VF PD maps that fell on abnormal (< 10%) OCT regions on the mGCIPL or RNFL probability maps. They noticed high levels of structure-function agreement, particularly when the 10-2 and 24-2 VF tests were combined (88.7% for early glaucoma; 2% for healthy). The agreement was 64.2% for early glaucoma and 4.4% for healthy eyes when only the 24-2 VF test was used, whereas the agreement was 77.4% for early glaucoma and 2.2% for healthy eyes using only the 10-2 VF test.

In a cross-sectional study, Hood *et al.* tested the hypothesis that a recently proposed PSD metric based upon the 24–2 VF test, as well as the PSD of the 10–2 VF, will miss central glaucomatous damage confirmed with an objective structure-function method.[5] In this study, a group of 70 early glaucoma eyes and a group of 45 healthy eyes were evaluated with 24-2 and 10-2 VFs and OCT scans twice within 4 weeks. The PSD based upon the central 12 points of the 24-2 VF test (PSD C24-2) was compared with the PSD of the 10-2 VF test (PSD 10-2).

To evaluate central defect in glaucoma eyes with normal PSD(C24-2) values, an analysis was done with a central defect reference standard, which was based upon an objective, topographic comparison between abnormal points on the 10-2 VF and OCT probability maps. In these 70 early glaucoma eyes, 44 had macular damage, but the PSD(C24-2) missed 27 (61%) of these and the PSD(10-2) missed 23 (52%). Hence, the results showed that the PSD(C24-2) as well as the standard PSD(10-2) miss a substantial number of eyes with macular damage, as defined above. Neither the PSD(C24-2) nor the PSD(10-2) are adequate metrics to identify early central defects. To identify both diffuse and local central defects caused by glaucoma, it is best to compare topographic agreement among OCT RGC layer and RNFL probability and thickness plots, as well as the topographic agreement between these OCT plots and VF loss on the 10-2 VF test.

De Moraes *et al.* showed that glaucoma staging systems based on the 24-2 VF test underestimate the severity of macular damage among patients with early glaucoma.[6] In their study of 57 eyes with early glaucoma, 48 had macular damage as defined by abnormal points (< 5% level) on the 10-2 VF test that topographically matched abnormal areas (< 5% level) of SD-OCT mRGC+ probability maps. Among eyes with macular damage, early defects were noticed in only 70% (95% CI, 55%–83%) by the Hodapp-Parrish-Anderson system, 81% (95% CI, 67%–91%) by the VFI system, and 68% (95% CI, 53%–81%) by the Brusini system. Chapter 4 discusses this particular study and related matters in detail.

3. A schematic model of glaucomatous damage to the macula

Hood[1] proposed a schematic model to understand glaucomatous damage to the macula. The macula is the central ±8° surrounding fixation and contains over 30% of RGCs. The schematic model suggests a map relating the locations of the RGCs on the retina to the regions around the optic disc where their axons enter. The RGC axons travel into the RNFL in bundles and enter the optic disc. The schematic model consists of 2 parts: a detailed map of the macular region describing the macular region, shown in Figure 3-1, and a comprehensive map of the retinal regions associated with the temporal half of the disc, as shown in Figure 3-2.

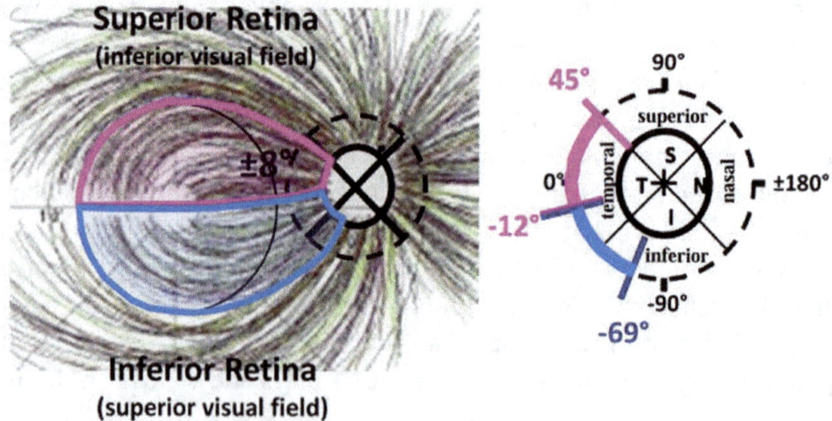

Fig. 3-1. The schematic model of the macula relates RGC axon locations to cpRNFL locations. This map of the macula relates the superior **(magenta)** and inferior **(light blue)** areas of the macula **(left)** to the associated regions of the optic disc (right). The dashed circle a circle that is 3.4 mm from the center of the disc, (dashed circle, right panel) is the location of the cpRNFL thickness plot. Reproduced from Hood.[1]

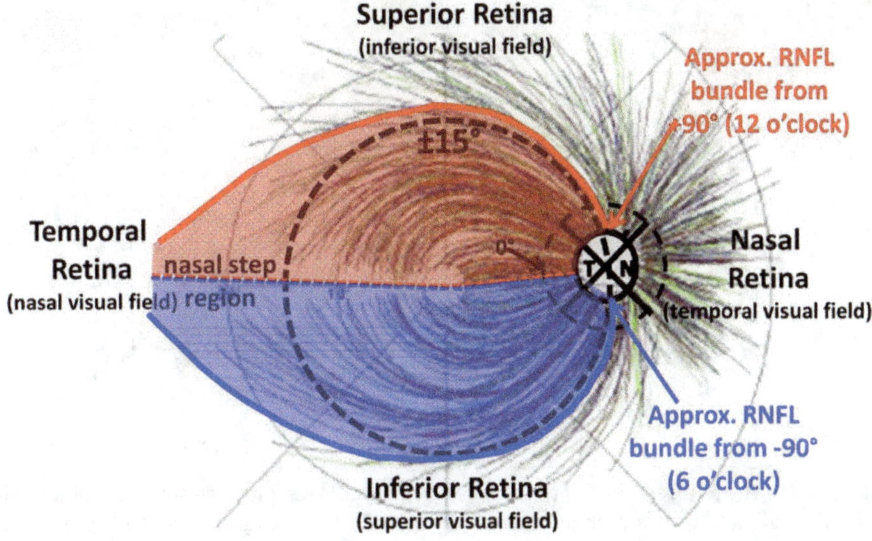

Fig. 3-2. The schematic model relates RGC axon locations to cpRNFL locations of the temporal half of the disc. The borders of the superior **(red)** and inferior **(blue)** regions of the retina supply retinal nerve fibers to the temporal half of the optic disc showing the course of the RNFL bundles related to the 12 o'clock **(red)** and 6 o'clock **(blue)** locations of the optic disc. This model suggests that the RGC axons from the retinal area within ±15° of the center of the fovea **(dashed black circle)** enter the temporal half of the optic disc. the axons of the RGCs within the red and blue borders enter the temporal half of the optic disc. RGC axons from the location of the retina labeled as the "nasal step" also enter the temporal half of the optic disc. This area of the retina is termed the "nasal step" because this location is associated with the nasal step defects seen on VFs. Reproduced from Hood.[1]

3.1 The nature of the damage to the macula and relatively vulnerable regions of the optic disc in early glaucomatous damage

A series of schematic models have been introduced to specify the relative vulnerability of optic disc local regions to early glaucomatous damage.[1] The schematic model in Figure 3-3 specifies the relative vulnerability of the local disc region to early glaucomatous damage. It is generally thought by Quigley and Green that local defects are common in the superior and inferior quadrants of the disc.[7] The temporal region of the optic disc is less vulnerable to glaucomatous damage than the inferior and superior quadrants, as documented by fundus photographs and OCT and HRT measurements.[8] Early damage is most common in the SVZ and IVZ. The SVZ and superior macular zone do not overlap. However, the IVZ and the inferior macular region overlap (Fig. 3-3). The region of overlap (Fig. 3-3A) is labeled

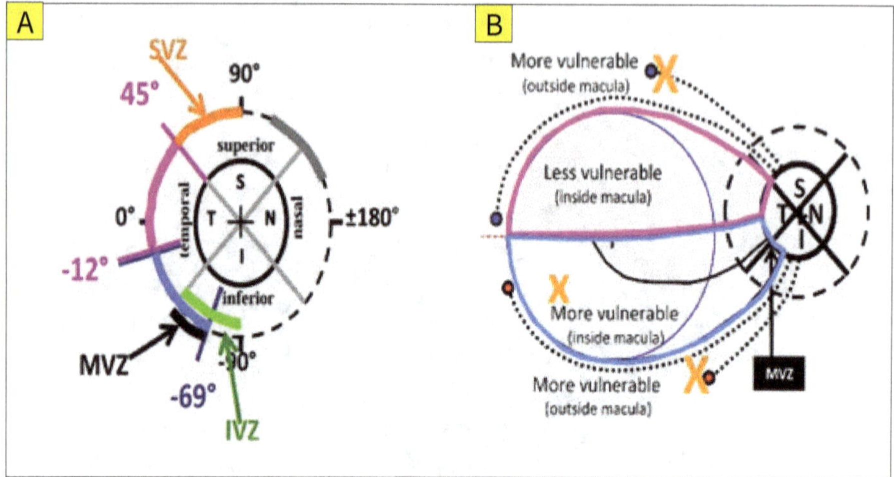

Fig. 3-3. (A) The temporal half of the disc has 2 vulnerable regions: The superior vulnerability zone (SVZ) and the inferior vulnerability zone (IVZ). The IVZ (green) overlaps the region of the cpRNFL (light blue) associated with the inferior macular retinal region. This region of overlap (black) is the macular vulnerability zone (MVZ). The SVZ (orange) does not overlap the region of the disc associated with the superior macular retinal region. **(B)** The retinal areas most vulnerable to glaucomatous damage include the area of the macula associated with the MVZ (white area within the light blue borders), along with the traditional arcuate region (large X) entering the SVZ and IVZ. Reproduced from Hood.[1]

as the MVZ. Therefore, the area of the retina more susceptible to glaucomatous damage includes the location of the macula associated with the MVZ along with the traditional arcuate zone entering the IVZ (Fig. 3-3B).

4. How local damage to the inferior retina includes both the macular and perimacular regions

The RNFL bundles in the superior macula from the RGCs in the central ± 8° enter the temporal quadrant of the disc, which is a region less at risk for glaucomatous damage. On the other hand, most of the RNFL bundles of the inferior macula enter the inferior quadrant of the disc, a region at high risk for glaucomatous damage. Only a small portion of the inferior RNFL bundles enter the temporal quadrant of the disc less susceptible to damage.

Early glaucoma generally affects areas both inside and outside of the macula. The schematic model provides a basis for understanding why both macular and perimacular damage is common in early glaucoma. The SVZ and the IVZ regions are only 45° wide, while the width of any local defects is generally more than 20°. Moreover, the MVZ comprises nearly 50% of the IVZ, with the rest of the IVZ devoted to the region outside the macula. Thus, local damage for the inferior retina. can include both the macular and perimacular regions.[1] The inferior macula is more susceptible to arcuate damage than the superior macula because of the region of the disc to which each is projected.

References

1. Hood DC. Improving our understanding, and detection, of glaucomatous damage: An approach based upon optical coherence tomography (OCT). Prog Retin Eye Res. 2017 Mar;57:46-75. https://doi.org/10.1016/j.preteyeres.2016.12.002

2. Chua J, Tan B, Ke M, et al. Diagnostic ability of individual macular layers by spectral-domain OCT in different stages of glaucoma. Ophthalmol Glaucoma. 2020 Sep-Oct;3(5):314-326. https://doi.org/10.1016/j.ogla.2020.04.003

3. Park HL, Lee J, Park CK. Visual field tests for glaucoma patients with initial macular damage: comparison between frequency-doubling technology and standard automated perimetry using 24-2 or 10-2 visual fields. J Glaucoma. 2018;27:627-634. https://doi.org/10.1097/IJG.0000000000000977

4. Hood DC, Tsamis E, Bommakanti NK, et al. Structure-function agreement is better than commonly thought in eyes with early glaucoma. Invest Ophthalmol Vis Sci. 2019;60:4241-4248. https://doi.org/10.1167/iovs.19-27920

5. Hood DC, Thenappan AA, Tsamis E, Liebmann JM, De Moraes CG. An evaluation of a new 24-2 metric for detecting early central glaucomatous damage. Am J Ophthalmol. 2021 Mar;223:119-128. https://doi.org/10.1016/j.ajo.2020.07.045

6. De Moraes CG, Sun A, Jarukasetphon R, et al. Association of macular visual field measurements with glaucoma staging systems. JAMA Ophthalmol. 2019;137(2):139-145. https://doi.org/10.1001/jamaophthalmol.2018.5398

7. Quigley HA, Green WR. The Histology of Human Glaucoma Cupping and Optic Nerve Damage: Clinicopathologic Correlation in 21 Eyes. Ophthalmology. 2020 Apr;127(4S): S45-S69. https://doi.org/10.1016/j.ophtha.2020.01.035

8. Hood DC, Raza AS, de Moraes CG, Johnson CA, Liebmann JM, Ritch R. The nature of macular damage in glaucoma as revealed by averaging optical coherence tomography data. Transl Vis Sci Technol. 2012 May 25;1(1):3. https://doi.org/10.1167/tvst.1.1.3

Chapter 4

The 24-2 visual field test underestimates central visual field defects

This chapter illustrates the limitations of the 24-2 VF test pattern to identify CVFDs, and highlights the shortcomings of existing standard metrics (MD, PSD, CC, and GHT) of the 24-2 test for detecting and interpreting CVFDs in early glaucoma.

1. Understanding the nature of glaucomatous macular damage from previous research

To understand the nature of glaucomatous damage, especially to the macula, a study used frequency domain OCT (fdOCT) macular cube scan to measure the local thickness of the RGC plus IPL.[1] RGC plus IPL can be expressed as the RGC+ layer. In this study, fdOCT macular and optic disc cube scans were obtained from 54 healthy eyes and 156 eyes with glaucomatous optic neuropathy. They categorized patients' eyes both by MD and hemifield classification using standard categories and 24-2 VFs. The study observed RGC+ and RNFL thinning on the average difference maps in the patient groups with VFs classified as normal. The thinning of RGC+ was mostly within the central 4 points of the 24-2 (6° grid) VF after correcting for RGC displacement. Therefore, RGC+ loss occurs in the central macula even in patients with VFs classified as normal, and the 6° grid (24-2) test pattern is not ideally designed to detect macular damage. Figure 4-1 presents a schematic model with the location of the VF test points. In Figure 4-2, the RGC+ thinning plot is superimposed on a fundus image.

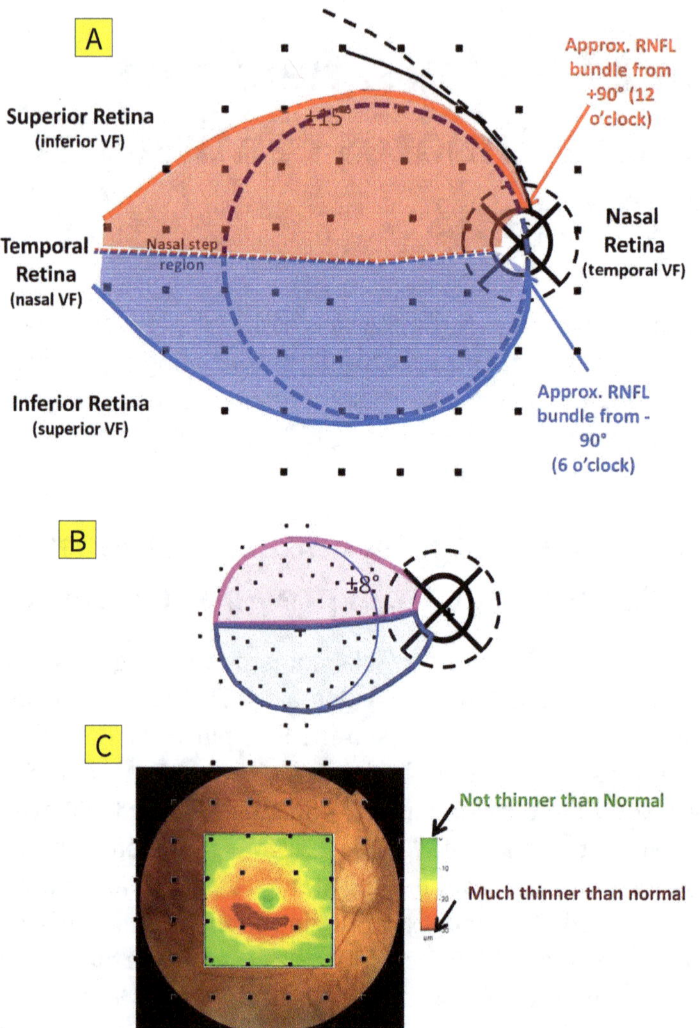

Fig. 4-1. The schematic model with the location of the VF test points. **(A)** Location of the 24-2 VF test points on the temporal half of the disc. The regions of the retina within the red and blue borders are the only regions associated with the temporal half of the disc. **(B)** Location of the 10-2 VF test points on the macular region. **(C)** A before fundus view with the RGC+ thinning map with the location of the 24-2VF test points. The MD of this VF < -5.5 dB. Reproduced from Hood.[2]

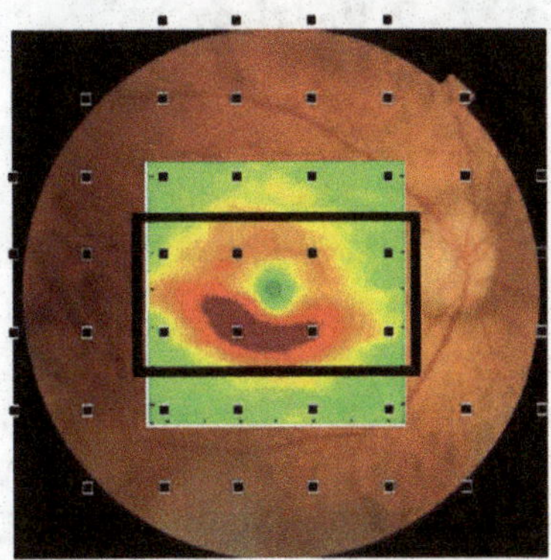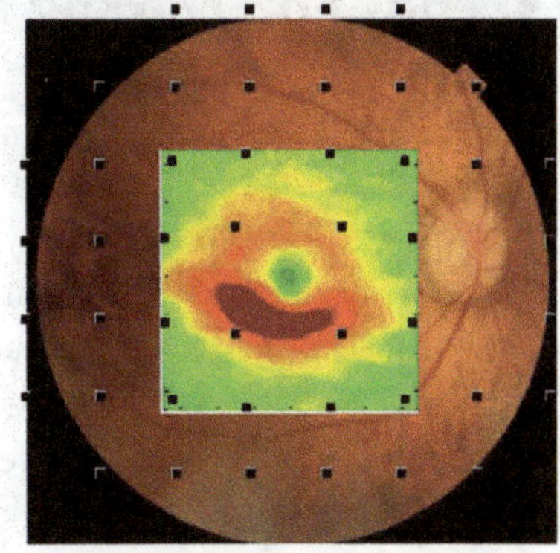

Fig. 4-2. Fundus image with the RGC+ thinning plot with 24-2 test locations. The RGC + thinning plot is superimposed on a fundus image. The 24-2 test locations are adjusted on this fundus view. **(Left)** The view without consideration of the displacement of the RGCs near the fovea and **(Right)** with consideration of the displacement. The MD of this VF is <-5.5 dB.[1] Only 4 points fall within the central 8°.[1] Reproduced from Hood *et al.*[1]

2. Glaucomatous macular damage is not represented by the OHTS

Patients with RGC+ damage in the central macula may present with a MD of 24-2 VF within normal limits, and their perimetric hemifields may be classified as normal by the existing guidelines. The OHTS classification includes 7 categories of VF, namely: Normal, Paracentral, Partial arcuate, Arcuate, Altitudinal, Nasal step, and Temporal wedge.[3] This classification system describes how nerve fiber bundle damage increases from paracentral to arcuate defects for early to moderate glaucomatous VF loss. However, the OHTS classification only includes classic patterns of VF defects and does not include VF loss caused by macular damage in glaucoma.[3] Specifically, the thinning of the macular RGC+ layer within the central points of the 24-2 test grid (Figs. 4-1C, 4-2) is not included in the category of VF defects introduced by OHTS. Therefore, this central macular damage is poorly represented in the categories of VF defects introduced by OHTS.

3. The shortcoming of the 24-2 VF test to recognize CVFDs

The 24-2 grid has 54 test locations to sample across the central 30° of the retina. Test point locations on the grid are separated by 6° vertically and horizontally. Thus, only 4 points fall within the central 8°, the region of the highest RGC density, where over 30% of RGCs are located. Therefore, this test pattern does not adequately sample the macular region in general, and defects near fixation are missed or underestimated with SAP 24-2 VFs, as previously discussed.[4-6] This is evident from fdOCT, when the displacement of the RGCs in the fovea is taken into consideration.[1]

If the central macular region had always been unaffected by glaucoma at its initial disease stages, this relatively poor sampling of the central 8° would not have been a major concern for a clinician. However, there is evidence that glaucoma patients may present with macular damage in the early disease stage, and even initial macular defects can occur in glaucoma patients as is evident from Figure 2-7 in Chapter 2.[7-9] Figure 4-3 presents representative cases where early glaucomatous defects near fixation were underestimated with a 24-2 VF test but detected with a 10-2 VF test.

3.1. Evidence found in robust studies

The following studies have observed that the 24-2 VF test can miss central damage in early glaucoma that is detected with the 10-2 VF test.

3.1.1. De Moraes et al.

This study compared the 24-2 and 10-2 VFs among 364 eyes with early glaucoma, 303 eyes of glaucoma suspects, 108 eyes with ocular hypertension (IOP > 22 mmHg), and 301 healthy controls.[4] A 24-2 VF was considered abnormal if there was a cluster of 3 contiguous depressed points within a hemifield with at least 1 at the < 1% level or 2 at the < 2% level (not necessarily involving the central 12 points). The same CC was used for the 10-2 VF. As per the CC, all but 26 early glaucoma eyes were detected as having abnormal 24-2 VFs. However, 16/26 eyes (61.5%) without an abnormal cluster on the 24-2 VF test pattern had an abnormal cluster on the 10-2 VF test pattern. Among the eyes with suspected glaucoma, 39.5% did not show any abnormal cluster in 24-2 VF test, while the same reported an abnormal cluster when tested with the 10-2 VF test. Similarly, among ocular hypertensive eyes, 28 out of 79 eyes (35.4%) were identified as normal on the 24-2 VF test, as per the CC. However, the same number of eyes were classified as abnormal on the 10-2 VF test. In comparison with these findings, only 14/303 healthy eyes (4.6%) with a normal 24-2 VF test had an abnormal cluster on the 10-2 VF test. This result suggests a specificity of 95% for the CC.

This study also compared the number of eyes without a central abnormality on the 24-2 VF, but had an abnormal 10-2 VF cluster. Central abnormality was defined as any of the 12 central points depressed at the ≤ 5% level. Among early glaucoma eyes, 60.6% of eyes were without any central abnormality on the 24-2 but had an abnormal cluster on the 10-2. Among glaucoma suspects, 36.7% of eyes showed normal central test points on the 24-2 but had an abnormal cluster defect on the 10-2. Similarly, in ocular hypertensive eyes, 34.2% of eyes with normal central 12 test points on the 24-2 showed abnormal cluster defects on the 10-2 test. This study also observed the presence of abnormal test points at the < 0.5% level on the TD or PD plot within the central 10°on the 24-2 test had a significant association with an abnormal 10-2 cluster (early glaucoma: OR, 7.52; 95% CI, 3.47–16.29; P < 0.001; glaucoma suspect: OR, 4.42; 95% CI, 1.20–16.18, P = 0.025).

3.1.2. Traynis et al.
This prospective observational cohort study evaluated the prevalence and nature of early glaucomatous visual field defects in the central 10° in glaucoma suspects and patients with early glaucoma.[6] One hundred eyes from 74 patients with early glaucoma were prospectively studied and tested with a 10-2 test. Reliable VF hemifields were classified as abnormal based on a CC, and abnormal 10-2 VFs were categorized based on the pattern of abnormal points.

They observed that 76 eyes had at least 1 hemifield defect on the 10-2 VF test. This finding showed that central defects are common among early glaucoma eyes. There appeared to be 53% abnormal 10-2 hemifields and 59% abnormal 24-2. Of the eyes with normal 24-2 hemifields, 16% were detected as abnormal when the 10-2 test was used and revealed that superior VF defects were deeper and closer to fixation than those in the inferior VF.

3.1.3. Roberti et al.

This study compared the detection rate of CVFD between the 30° Octopus G1 program (Dynamic strategy) and the HFA 10-2 SITA-Standard test in early glaucoma eyes not showing any CVFD on the HFA 24-2 SITA-Standard test.[10] They observed that both HFA 10-2 and Octopus G1 programs found CVFDs not detected with the HFA 24-2 test. A CVFD was present in 80.4% of eyes on HFA 10-2 test and in 56% on Octopus G1 tests ($P = 0.002$).

3.1.4. Tomairek et al.

This study evaluated the role of 10-2 VF test in different stages of glaucoma. They observed low agreement between the 10-2 VF test and the central 10° points on the 24-2 VF test among 47 early glaucoma eyes.[11] This study inferred that a 10-2 test could confirm a glaucoma diagnosis missed by a 24-2 test in glaucoma suspects. In early glaucoma, they observed that a 10-2 test was a beneficial addition to the 24-2 test for precise measurement of the MD and detection of defects within central 10° missed by the 24-2 test.

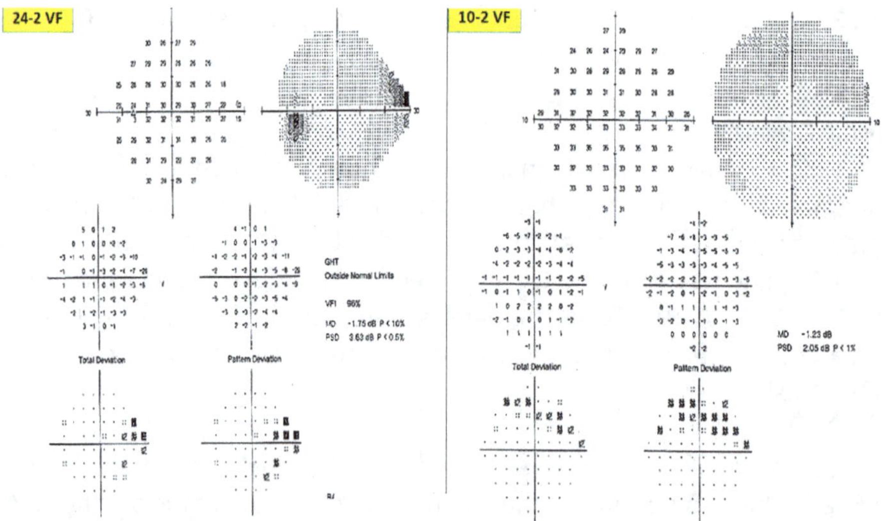

Fig. 4-3. Early glaucomatous defects near fixation were underestimated with a 24-2 VF test. This patient's early glaucomatous superior nasal defect in the left eye is evident in both TD and PD probability plots. However, there is an isolated single abnormal 24-2 VF point depressed at $P < 5\%$ in the central 5° in the superior nasal hemifield. When the same patient was tested on the same day with a 10-2 test pattern, the central field defect was noticed on 10-2 VF. The 10-2 test displayed an arcuate-like PFS on both probability plots of the 10-2 test pattern . That PFS was missed by the 24-2 VF test.

3.1.5. Grillo et al.

The purpose of this study was to determine the extent to which the 24-2 VF misses macular damage confirmed with both 10-2 VF and OCT scans and to evaluate the patterns of damage missed.[5] The investigators noted that 24-2 VF metrics missed eyes with confirmed glaucomatous macular damage or CVFDs and that such eyes may be classified as normal based on the 24-2 VF alone.

4. Existing standard metrics for detecting VF defects in glaucoma

The most common clinical paradigm for diagnosing glaucoma includes a VF test with a 6° test grid (24-2/30-2 test pattern) and an OCT scan of the optic disc (Fig. 4-4).[12] The assessment of these test results depends on quantitative metrics. For the VF, standard quantitative metrics are the MD, PSD, and GHT of the VF; for OCT, metrics are the global or quadrant cpRNFL thickness/probabilities of the OCT disc scan for detecting and comparing abnormal VF and OCT scans.

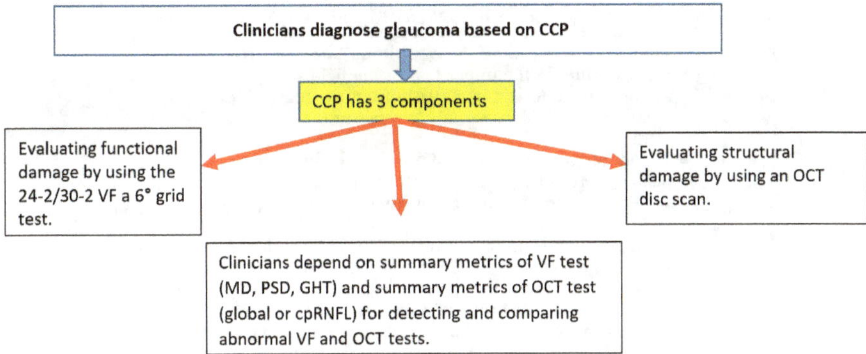

Fig. 4-4. The common clinical paradigm (CCP) for diagnosing glaucoma.

5. Limitations of summary metrics of the VF test to detect a CVFD on 24-2 VF

In the following sections, we will enumerate the limitations of 24-2 metrics namely, the GHT, MD, and CC for recognizing early glaucomatous functional loss within the central 10° of a 24-2 VF as indicated by current research.[5]

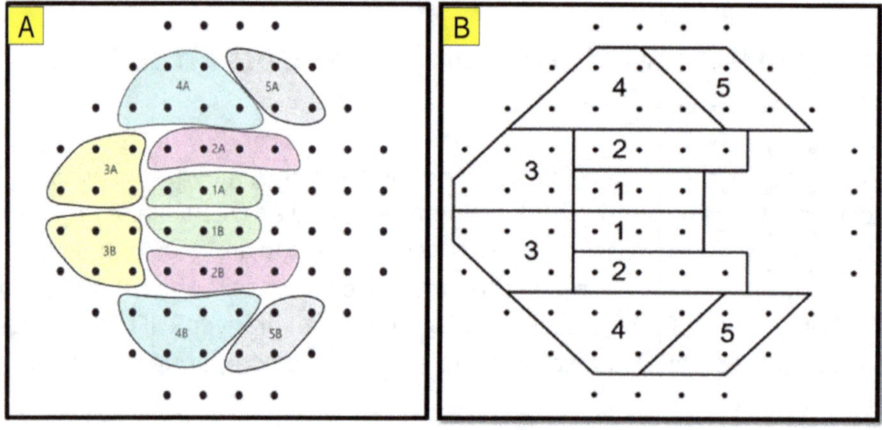

C
Glaucoma Hemifield Test Classification

- Outside Normal Limits: Sensitivities in one or more of the five zones in the upper half of the field are significantly different (p < 0.01) from the sensitivities measured in the corresponding zones in the lower half of the field.
- Borderline: the sensitivity differences between zone pairs are greater than those seen in most normal subjects (p < 0.03), but do not reach the level required for the previous message.
- General Depression of Sensitivity: The point with the seventh highest deviation from normal is under the 0.5% probability level.
- Abnormally High Sensitivity: The best point locations are over the 0.5% probability level.
- Within Normal Limits: None of the above significance limits are reached.
- The dual statement "Borderline + General Reduction of Sensitivity" appears when a significant diffuse sensitivity depression is combined with an up-down difference at the p < 0.03 level.

Fig. 4-5. (A) The GHT compares PD probability scores in 5 zones in the upper field with corresponding scores in the mirror image lower field. Reproduced from Chakravarti *et al.*[13] **(B)** The GHT uses a subset (22 test locations in the superior/inferior hemifields) of the 24-2 test pattern. Reproduced from Chakravarti.[13] **(C)** The 5 possible outcomes of the GHT results. Reproduced from Brusini and Johnson.[14]

> **Anderson-Patella's criteria to detect early glaucomatous VF damage on HFA 30-2/24-2 program:**
>
> 1)In a location typical for glaucoma damage, a cluster of >3 non-edge points depressed at P<5% and one of which at P<1%, in the pattern deviation plot in a single hemifield (superior/inferior);
>
> 2) GHT result outside of normal limits;
>
> 3) Abnormal PSD with P<5%
>
> 1. Meeting any 1 of these 3 criteria is sufficient for diagnosis
> 2. Confirmation by consistent findings on 2 consecutive fields

Fig. 4-6. Anderson-Patella's criteria to detect early glaucomatous VF damage on HFA 30-2/24-2 VF.

5.1. The accuracy of the GHT is questioned in detecting early glaucoma

GHT hemifield clusters (Fig. 4-5A, 4-5B) offer high sensitivity and specificity for detecting early glaucomatous VF changes and provide early discrimination of VF loss than other global indices (MD, PSD) especially when repeated measures show consistent asymmetry. The GHT interpretation Outside Normal Limits is considered the single most efficient method of VF interpretation; it is claimed to be the most accurate among the 3 minimum criteria of the Hodapp-Parrish-Anderson criteria (Fig. 4-6) for diagnosing early glaucomatous damage.[15] However, GHT is not as sensitive in recognizing early glaucomatous loss as has been previously thought.[13,16]

5.2. GHT Analysis

1. The GHT utilizes a subset of 22 test locations in the superior/inferior hemifields (Fig. 4-5A, 4-5B).
2. These 22 test locations in each hemifield are divided into 5 zones based on the mapping of retinal locations to the ONH.
3. The GHT compares PD probability scores in 5 zones in the superior hemifield with corresponding scores in the mirror image of the inferior hemifield.
4. The GHT assigns a score to each test point based on values presented in the PD probability maps and then calculates a sum for each sector (Fig. 4-5C).
5. GHT is directed primarily at diagnosing glaucomatous VF loss, and not other diseases.

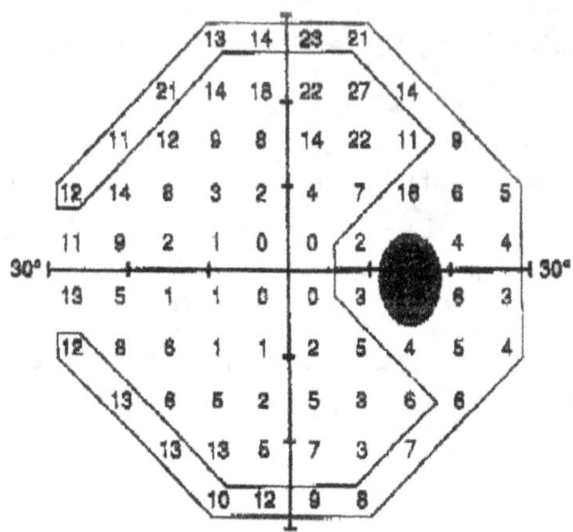

Fig. 4-7. GHT test locations within and outside the enclosure map. In GHT, an irregular enclosure map represents test loci not included in the 5 GHT mirror-image zones. Reproduced from Zalta.[16]

5.3. GHT interpretations are subject to the following limitations

- The 5 GHT mirror image comparison zones are designed to exclude all test loci adjacent to the blind spot. The GHT zones also ignore all loci in the temporal step area and all loci between 25° and 30°, except for a single test point immediately adjacent to the nasal raphe at 27° eccentricity (Fig. 4-7).[13,16]

- The GHT underappreciates test points to detect real nasal depressions, real temporal steps, and real edge defects. Hence, there is a risk that early loss could cut across the GHT sector boundaries and fail to display significant abnormality in either sector.

- The specificity of GHT is approximately 94% when Borderline findings are treated as being Within Normal Limits, and approximately 84% when Borderline findings are considered Outside Normal Limits.

- Some investigators consider that the Within Normal Limits GHT interpretation may be a flaw in GHT analysis (Fig. 4-8A).[13] GHT Within Normal Limits is often unable to identify well-established, reproducible glaucomatous early defects in PD probability plots. According to some researchers, the GHT Borderline is also considered a flaw of GHT analysis that fails to recognize reproducible VF defects in PD probability maps (Fig. 4-8B).[13,16]

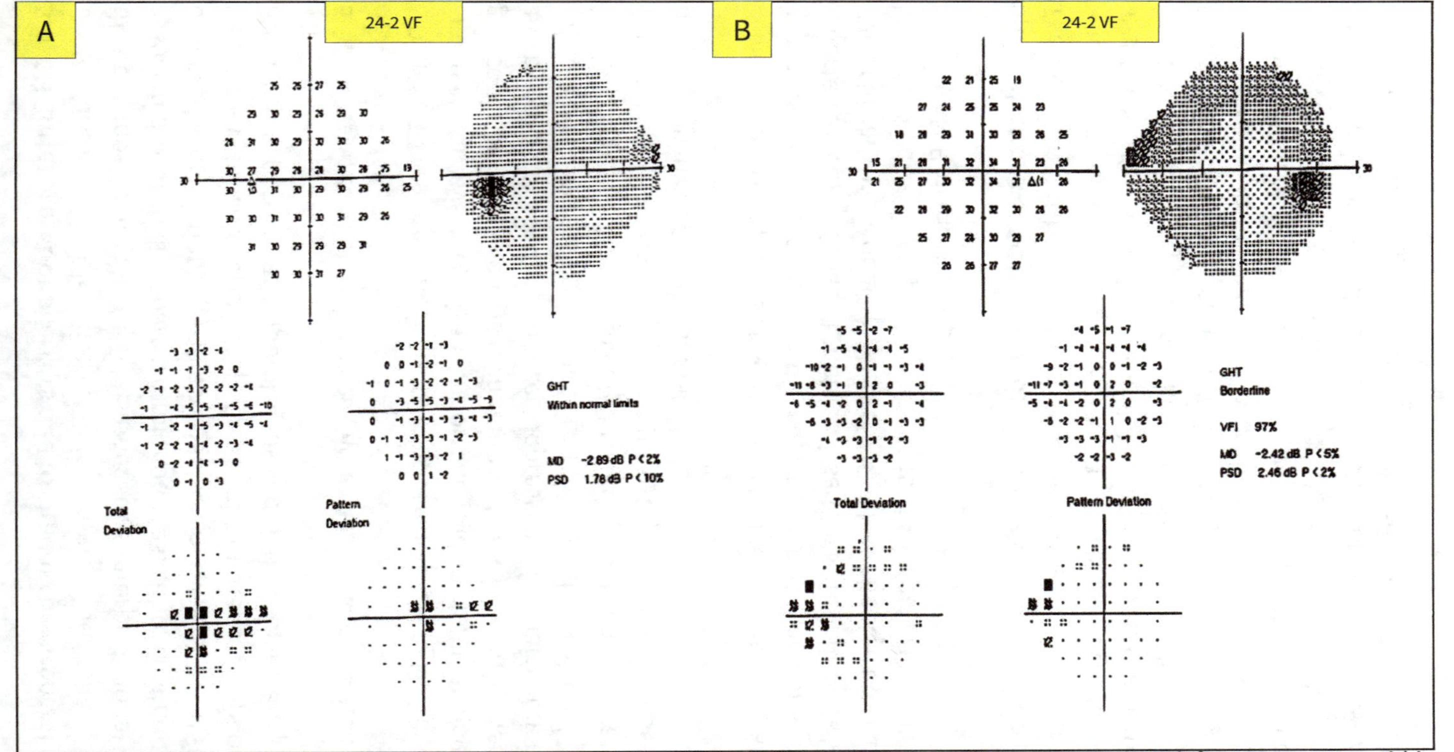

Fig. 4-8. Misinterpretation of early glaucomatous VF defects by GHT. **(A)** In this 24-2 VF, the earliest glaucomatous defects are present within the central° 10 and a nasal defect on both the TD and PD probability plots. However, GHT interprets this 24-2 VF as Within Normal Limits (WNL) despite the presence of a glaucomatous defect as PFS and PNS. **(B)** Another 24-2 VF is interpreted by the GHT as Borderline despite the presence of a real scotoma in the nasal field.

5.4. GHT interpretational errors due to shallow paracentral defects

On the accuracy of GHT interpretation, some reports have pointed out that the most common GHT false negative interpretational errors were associated with shallow paracentral scotomas. Other common errors were observed with inferior edge defects (test loci between 25° and 30° eccentricity), shallow arcuate, and nasal depressions or steps. Errors occurred less frequently in detecting temporal steps and shallow biarcuate scotomas.[13,16]

5.5. Limitations of global indices (MD and PSD) to evaluate central defects

MD and PSD are the 2 most popular global indices used in clinical practice and have always played an important role in summarizing VF loss in glaucoma, although both have limitations. MD is affected by media opacities and by other causes of generalized depression of visual function in addition to glaucoma. Increasing cataracts can mislead the clinician by suggesting a high progression rate. Again, MD value improves after cataract surgery. Thus, by applying preoperative and postoperative MD values, glaucoma progression may be underestimated.

More importantly, MD is very weakly centered and weighed, and therefore is not very well correlated to the patient's visual function. A recent study reported that the MD 24-2 VF metric missed 34% of confirmed glaucomatous CVFDs in early glaucoma on 24-2VF.[5] PSD is less affected by media opacities but has the disadvantage that it erroneously displays improvement as the severity of VF loss increases.

5.6 Limitations of CC for detecting central defects in early glaucoma

The CC metric of the 24-2 VF is designed to detect local damage. As per existing guidelines, the CC is defined as 3 neighboring points at 5%, 5%, and 1% or 5%, 2%, and 2% probability or worse within a hemifield on TD or PD plots, with only 1 point allowed on the edge of the 24-2 VF. Previous research indicates the imprecise guidelines for CC for evaluating abnormal points located in the central 5° with depressed sensitivity (from -4 dB to -12 dB).[13] Therefore, 24-2 VF with early glaucomatous central defects may be underdiagnosed due to the lack of proper guidelines for identifying an abnormal cluster. It is not necessary that a cluster should always be formed by 3 adjacent depressed test points in the hemifield. Precisely for this very reason, paracentral and central scotomas often remain undiagnosed or underdiagnosed.

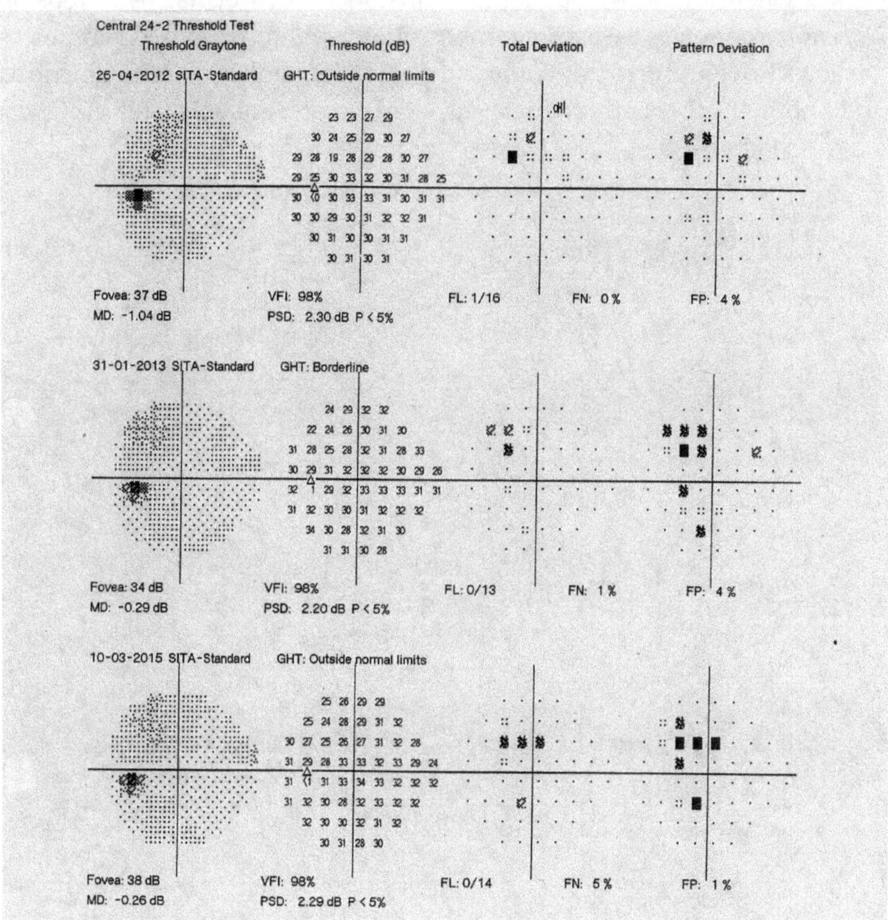

Fig. 4-9. (A) The overview printout shows a 50-year-old male patient presenting a small cluster of defective points in the same area on 24-2 VF on repeated examinations from 2012 to 2015. The 3 fields shown on this page show a typical transition over a 3-year period from a very early VF defect to a well-established glaucomatous defect. Test-retest variability is increased in the area that finally becomes definitely abnormal. The GHT misinterprets the second VF on the overview as a Borderline defect.

Without proper guidelines, repeated, confirmatory findings often are needed before a diagnosis of manifest glaucoma can be made with certainty. Hence, when following a patient, for instance, with ocular hypertension with apparent early defects, clinicians often label these early VF losses as shallow VF defects that may come and go. Consequently, patients' diagnosis and treatment decisions are delayed. Here we present an example of such a case in Figure 4-9.

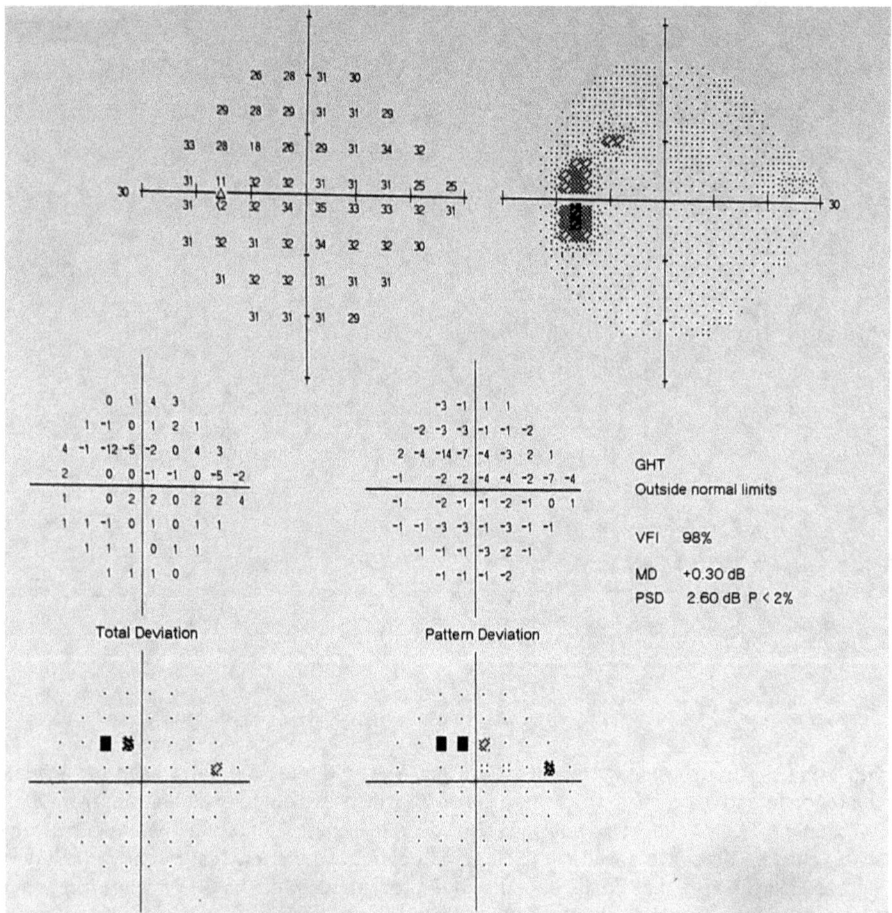

Fig. 4-9. (B) His 24-2 VF, in 2016, showed early glaucomatous paracentral defects in the TD and PD probability plots but the MD value (+ 0.30 dB) is better than the MD values recorded in VFs from 2012 to 2015 in the overview printout. However, the VFI retains the same percentage (98%) in the overview printout and this VF report. Therefore, the global indices underappreciate the severity of the paracentral defects.

A recent study by Grillo *et al.* reported that 59 eyes with glaucomatous macular defects were confirmed based on 10-2 VF and OCT macular scans. Of those 59 eyes, 52.5% of eyes were missed (false negative) by 1 or more 24-2 VF metrics.[5] CC, the most sensitive 24-2 VF metric, missed 12% of the eyes with confirmed macular damage. MD, the least sensitive 24-2 VF metric, missed 34% of eyes with such defect.[5] Grillo *et al.* concluded, that for detecting macular damage (CVFD) reliably with perimetry, either the 10-2 VF test or a modified 24-2 VF test is crucial.

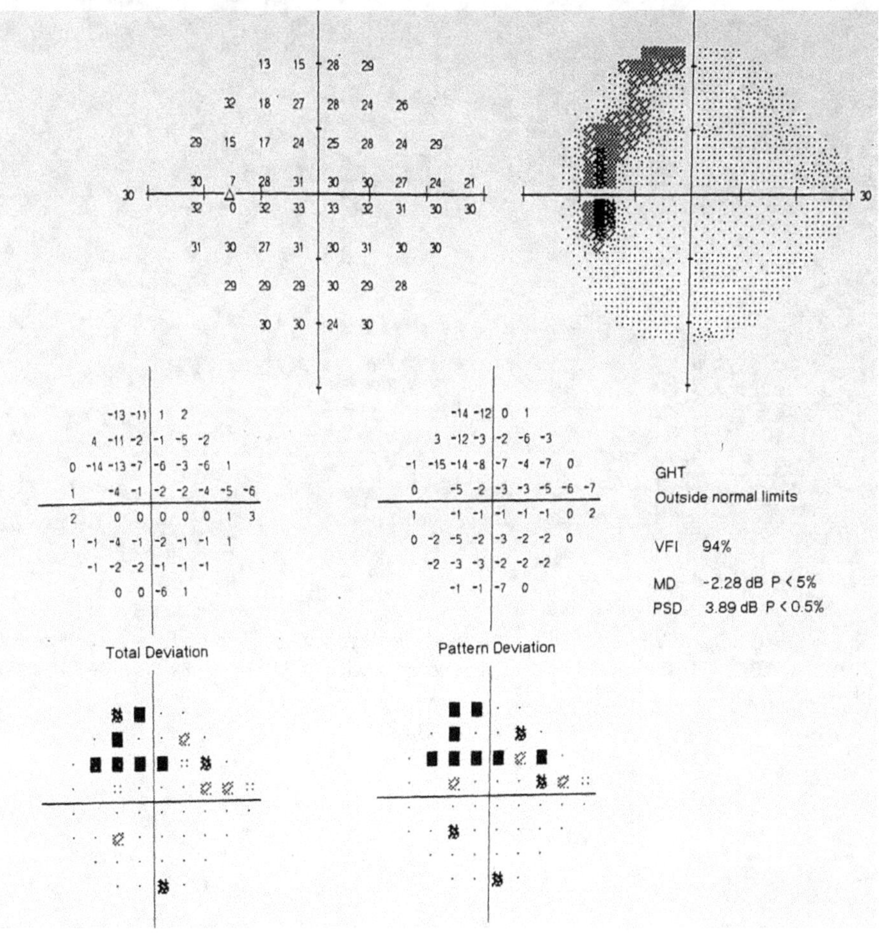

Fig. 4-9. (C) Deterioration of his initial VF defect in the same eye was recorded in 2019 with VFI 94%, MD -2.28 dB, and PSD 3.89 dB.

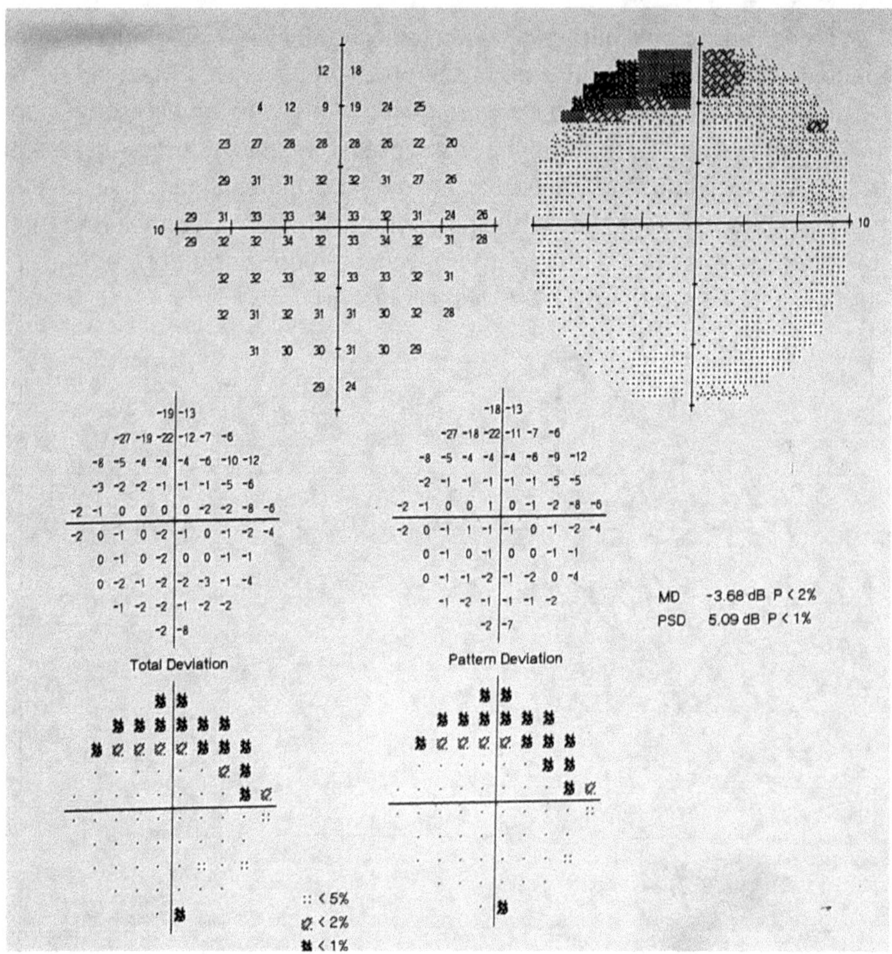

Fig. 4-9. (D) Central VF defect in the patient's left eye was confirmed by a 10-2 VF test in 2020. The 10-2 VF test showed an arcuate scotoma with an MD of -3.68 dB and PSD of 5.09 dB.

References

1. Hood DC, Raza AS, de Moraes CG, Johnson CA, Liebmann JM, Ritch R. The nature of macular damage in glaucoma as revealed by averaging optical coherence tomography data. Transl Vis Sci Technol. 2012 May 25;1(1):3. https://doi.org/10.1167/tvst.1.1.3

2. Hood DC. Improving our understanding, and detection, of glaucomatous damage: An approach based upon optical coherence tomography (OCT). Prog Retin Eye Res. 2017 Mar; 57:46-75. https://doi.org/10.1016/j.preteyeres.2016.12.002

3. Keltner JL, Johnson CA, Cello, KE, et al. Ocular Hypertension Treatment Study Group. Classification of visual field abnormalities in the ocular hypertension treatment study. Arch Ophthalmol. 2003 May; 121 (5): 643-50. https://doi.org/10.1001/archopht.121.5.643

4. De Moraes CG, Hood DC, Thenappan A, et al. 24-2 visual fields miss central defects shown on 10-2 tests in glaucoma suspects, ocular hypertensives, and early glaucoma. Ophthalmology. 2017;124:1449-1456. https://doi.org/10.1016/j.ophtha.2017.04.021

5. Grillo LM, Wang DL, Ramachandran R, et al. The 24-2 visual field test misses central macular damage confirmed by the 10-2 visual field test and optical coherence tomography. Transl Vis Sci Technol. 2016;5:15. https://doi.org/10.1167/tvst.5.2.15

6. Traynis I, De Moraes CG, Raza AS, et al. Prevalence and nature of early glaucomatous defects in the central 10° of the visual field. JAMA Ophthalmol. 2014;132:291-297. https://doi.org/10.1001/jamaophthalmol.2013.7656

7. Aulhorn E, Harms M. Early visual field defects in glaucoma. In: Leydhecker W, editor. Glaucoma, Tutzing Symposium. Basel: Karger; 1967. p. 151-186. https://doi.org/10.1159/000389404

8. Aulhorn E, Karmeyer H. Frequency distribution in early glaucomatous visual field defects. Doc Ophthalmol Proc Series. 1977;14:17-83.

9. Drance SM. The early field defects in glaucoma. Invest Ophthalmol. 1969;8(1):84-91.

10. Roberti G, Manni G, Riva I, et al. Detection of central visual field defects in early glaucomatous eyes: Comparison of Humphrey and Octopus perimetry. PLoS One. 2017 Oct 27;12(10) https://doi.org/10.1371/journal.pone.0186793

11. Tomairek RH, Aboud SA, Hassan M, Mohamed AH. Studying the role of 10-2 visual field test in different stages of glaucoma. Eur J Ophthalmol. 2020;30(4):706-713. https://doi.org/10.1177/1120672119836904

12. Hood DC, De Moraes CG. Challenges to the common clinical paradigm for diagnosis of glaucomatous damage with OCT and visual fields. Invest Ophthalmol Vis Sci. 2018;59(2):788-791. https://doi.org/10.1167/iovs.17-23713

13. Chakravarti T. Assessing precision of Hodapp-Parrish-Anderson criteria for staging early glaucomatous damage in an ocular hypertension cohort: A retrospective study.

Asia Pac J Ophthalmol (Phila). 2017 Jan-Feb;6(1):21-27. https://doi.org/10.1097/APO.0000000000000201

14. Brusini P, Johnson CA. Staging functional damage in glaucoma: review of different classification methods. Surv Ophthalmol. 2007 Mar-Apr;52(2):156-79. https://doi.org/10.1016/j.survophthal.2006.12.008

15. Asman P, Heijl A. Evaluation of methods for automated Hemifield analysis in perimetry. Arch Ophthalmol. 1992;110(6):820-826. https://doi.org/10.1001/archopht.1992.01080180092034

16. Zalta AH. Limitations of the glaucoma hemifield test in identifying early glaucomatous field loss. Ann Ophthalmol. 2000;32:33-45. https://doi.org/10.1007/s12009-000-0010-9

Chapter 5

Current glaucoma staging systems underestimate disease severity in eyes with central visual field defects

This chapter elucidates how current glaucoma staging systems based on 24-2 or 30-2 SAP results underestimate the disease severity of glaucoma patients with CVFDs (*i.e.*, glaucomatous macular damage). In this chapter, we present commonly used classification systems and explain how they underestimate the severity of CVFDs in early glaucoma.

1. Classification of glaucomatous functional damage severity

Presently, more than 20 severity classifications are available for quantifying glaucomatous VF damage and few of these staging systems take into account the presence of central VF damage as a sign of more severe disease.

Recently, De Moraes *et al.* verified the precision of current glaucoma staging systems in patients with early glaucoma and with glaucomatous CVFDs. They included 57 eyes with early glaucoma (MD <-6 dB on 24-2VF) and applied Hodapp-Parrish-Anderson (HPA), Glaucoma Visual Field Staging System (GVFSS), and Brusini staging systems for evaluating disease severity and compare such VFs.[1] The study found that current glaucoma staging systems underrate glaucoma severity in eyes with central damage, for these grading systems are based on 24-2 or 30-2 SAP results and these tests do not adequately evaluate macular function.[1]

2. Glaucoma severity staging systems commonly used in clinical practice and research

2.1. Hodapp-Parrish-Anderson criteria

The Hodapp-Parrish-Anderson (HPA) criteria[2] uses 2 criteria for staging. The first criterion counts the overall damage extent, calculated using both the MD value and the number of depressed points in the Humphrey Statpac-2 PD probability plot. The second criterion is based on the loss of threshold sensitivity within the central 5° of the VF. Table 5-1 presents the HPA classification for early, moderate, and severe VF defects.

Table 5-1. The HPA criteria

Criteria for early defect
• Mean deviation ≤ -6 dB on PD plot
• < 25% of points depressed less than the 5% level and < 15% of points depressed less than the 1% level
• No point within the central 5° with sensitivity < 15 dB
Criteria for moderate defect
• MD > -6 dB but < -12 dB on PD plot
• < 50% of points depressed less than the 5% level and < 25% of points depressed less than the 1% level
• No point within the central 5° with sensitivity < 0 dB
• Only 1 hemifield containing a point with sensitivity < 15 dB within 5° of fixation
Criteria for severe defect (any of the following results):
• MD > -12 dB on PD plot
• > 50% of points depressed below the 5% level or > 25% of points depressed below the 1% level
• Any point within the central 5° with sensitivity ≤ 0 dB
• Both hemifields containing point(s) with sensitivity < 15 dB within 5° of fixation

2.2. VFI system

The VFI system[3] classifies VF results according to VFI values, whereby:

- Early: Values > 91%
- Moderate: Values between 78% and 91%
- Severe: Values < 78%

2.3. Brusini Glaucoma Staging System 2

The Brusini Glaucoma Staging System 2 (GSS2)[4] is based on a chart that plots global metrics from the HFA or the Octopus perimeter. The HFA metrics of MD and PSD are plotted on the x-axis and y-axis, respectively (Fig. 5-1 and table 5-2). The solid curves are the borders between the stages of the system. The intersection between MD and PSD values defines whether the eye has localized, generalized, or mixed defects, as well as its stage, ranging from 0 (less severe) to 4 (more severe).

2.4. MD staging system

The modified MD staging system proposed by Mills *et al.*[5,6] is based solely on the MD values of the 24-2 or 30-2 VFs, whereby:

- Early glaucoma: better than -6.00 dB
- Moderate glaucoma: -6.01 to -12.00 dB
- Advanced glaucoma: -12.01 to -22.00 dB
- Severe glaucoma: -22.01 dB or worse

2.5. Aulhorn and Karmeyer's classification

Aulhorn and Karmeyer classify the extent of VF defects into the following stages:[7]

- Stage I: Only relative defects
- Stage II: Spot-like, stroke-like, or arcuate absolute defects, having no connection to the blind spot
- Stage III: Arcuate absolute defects already connected to the blind spot, with or without a nasal breakthrough into the periphery
- Stage IV: Extensive ring-shaped or half-ring-shaped defects, with a central island of sensitivity maintained
- Stage V: Central island collapse, with only the temporal VF area remaining

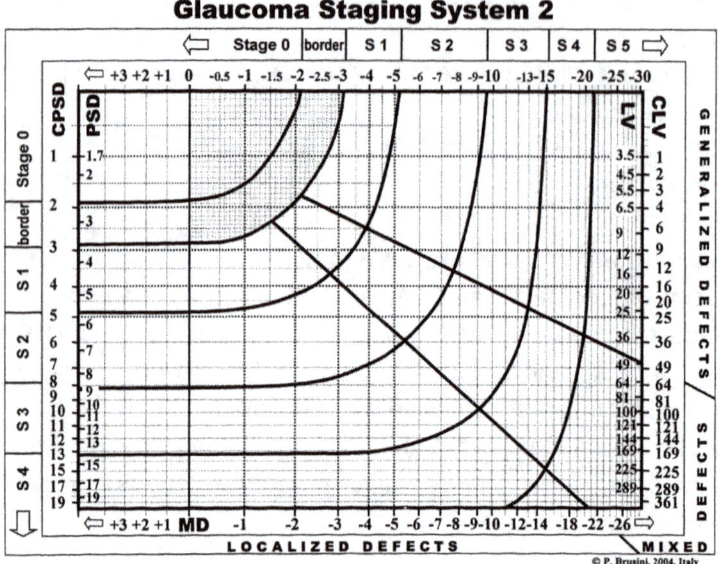

Fig. 5-1. Brusini's GSS2 is based on MD and CPSD values, where the intersection of the MD and PSD values defines both the stage and type of defect. CPSD: corrected PSD. Reproduced from Brusini *et al.*[4]

Table 5-2. Classification based on MD and corrected PSD values by Brusini *et al.*

Stage	Parameters
0	Both MD and CPSD within normal limits
1	MD between -3 and -5 dB and CPSD ≤ 3 dB or MD < -3 dB and CPSD between 3 and 5 dB or Both MD and CPSD between -3 and -5 dB
2	MD > -5 dB and < 8 dB and CPSD < 8 dB or MD < -3 dB and CPSD > 5 dB and < 8dB
3	MD between -8 and -12 dB or CPSD ≥ 8 dB
4	MD ≥ -12 dB and < -20 dB
5	MD ≥ -20 dB

CPSD: Corrected PSD

Modified from Brusini *et al.*[4]

2.6. Advanced Glaucoma Intervention Study scoring system

The Advanced Glaucoma Intervention Study (AGIS) scoring system assigns[8] VF scores divided into 5 stages (Fig. 5-2 and Table 5-3) whereby:

- Score 0–5: Normal
- Score 1–5: Mild damage
- Score 6–11: Moderate damage
- Score 12–17: Severe damage
- Score 18–20: End-stage

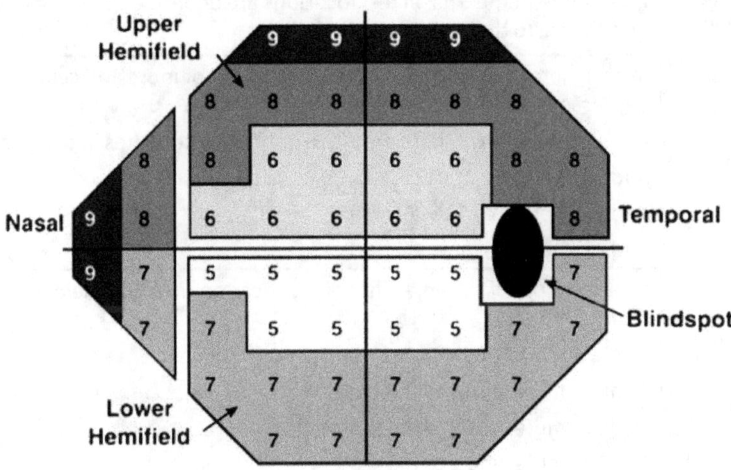

Fig. 5-2. AGIS Visual Field Test Scoring. Reproduced from Advanced Glaucoma Intervention Study.[8]

Table 5-3. The AGIS score for evaluating the severity of glaucomatous damage

The AGIS score ranges from 0 to 20, and it is obtained as follows:	
Nasal defect, nasal step, hemifield defect	A cluster of 3 or more adjacent depressed test locations among the 6 test sites in the nasal field constitutes a *nasal defect*. The cluster may cross the horizontal midline.
	One or more depressed test locations in the nasal field, either above or below the horizontal midline, in the absence of depression of any of the 3 test locations on the opposite side of the horizontal midline, constitutes a *nasal step*.
	A cluster of 3 depressed sites in a hemifield constitutes a *hemifield defect*. More than 1 cluster of depressed sites may occur in a hemifield.
Points are awarded to the score as follows:	For a nasal defect or nasal step, add 1 to the score.
	If 4 or more of the 6 nasal test locations are depressed 12 dB or more, add 1 more to the score.
	In each hemifield with 1 or more clusters of 3 or more adjacent depressed test locations (hemifield defects):
	Add 1 to the score if there are 3 to 5 depressed test sites in the clusters.
	Add 2 if there are 6 to 12.
	Add 3 if there are 13 to 20.
	Add 4 if there are more than 20.
	If half or more of the adjacent defect, locations in a hemifield are depressed:
	28 dB, add 5 to the score.
	24 dB or more, add 4 to the score.
	20 dB or more, add 3 to the score.
	16 dB or more, add 2 to the score.
	12 dB or more, add 1 to the score.
	This series of steps may add as much as 5 to the score for each hemifield containing a deep defect.
	If a hemifield lacks a cluster of 3 adjacent depressed test sites, but contains at least 2 adjacent depressed sites of which one is depressed 12 dB or more, add 1 to the score.

3. Glaucoma staging systems count the loss of threshold sensitivity within the central 5° of the VF

The HPA classification system and the grading system proposed by Mills *et al.*, similar to the HPA method, take into consideration the proximity of defect(s) to fixation. Another grading system suggested by the University of São Paulo (Brazil) is the Glaucoma Visual Field Staging System, in which qualitative and quantitative characteristics of the VF defect are described.[9] This system considers the location of the defect in 3 categories: VF defect inside the central 5°; VF defect inside the central 10° but outside the central 5°; VF defect outside the central 10°.

4. Representative cases that explain how commonly used classification systems underrate the severity of early glaucoma

Two representative cases (Figs. 5-3, 5-4) describe how the current clinical paradigm for glaucoma care, based on 24-2 VFs, is insufficient for accurately diagnosing glaucoma and determining its severity and effect on QoL. Clinicians are still over-dependent on summary metrics derived from VFs (*e.g.*, MD, PSD, and VFI) and also from high-resolution spectral domain OCT scans. Again, test-retest variability is greater in VF metrics than in OCT metrics, and VF metrics are more influenced by disease severity.[10,11]

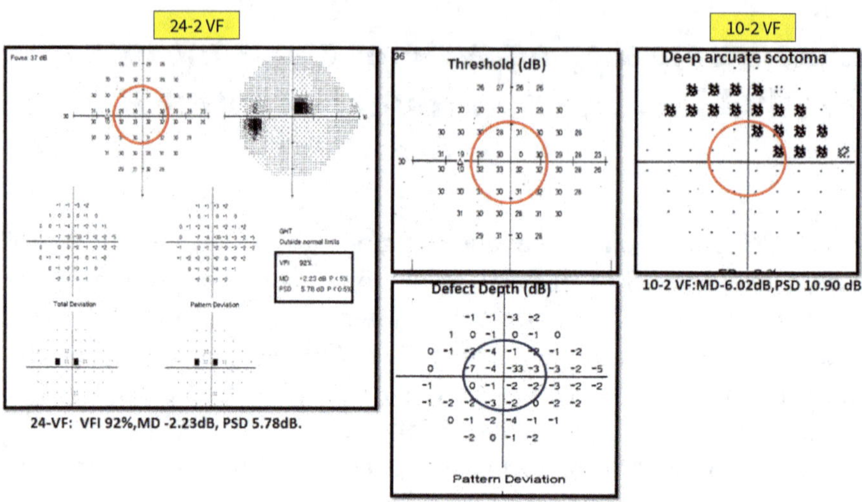

Fig. 5-3. Disease severity in glaucomatous eyes with CVFDs in the early disease stage is underestimated by 24-2 VF testing. This VF of a 40-year-old male patient having NTG presented with an abnormal 24-2 VF point at the superior nasal location in the central 5° and 1 abnormal paracentral point within the central 10° in his left eye. Both abnormal points were depressed $P < 0.5\%$ and were uniformly depressed at -33 dB on the TD and PD plots; threshold sensitivity was also maximally low at 0 dB. Staging systems based on summary metrics (*e.g.* MD, PSD, and VFI) such as the modified MD staging system proposed by Miller *et al.*, the VFI system, and Brusini's GSS2, classified this VF as having an early disease or Borderline disease. AGIS scoring classified this VF as having a moderate defect. As the HPA system takes into account the presence of abnormalities within the central 5° of the 24-2 grid, this VF was classified as having a severe stage. Finally, this eye was tested with a 10-2 VF test grid, which displayed deep arcuate defect with worse MD (-6.0 dB) and PSD (10.9 dB) than the initial defect in the 24-2 VF (MD of −2.2 dB and PSD of 5.7 dB). A detailed image of the points within the central 10°, the threshold value of abnormal points **(red circle)**, and defect depth **(blue circle)** are highlighted. In the 10-2 plot **(extreme right)**, the points within 10° of fixation are outlined with a red circle. Modified from Chakravarti *et al.*[12]

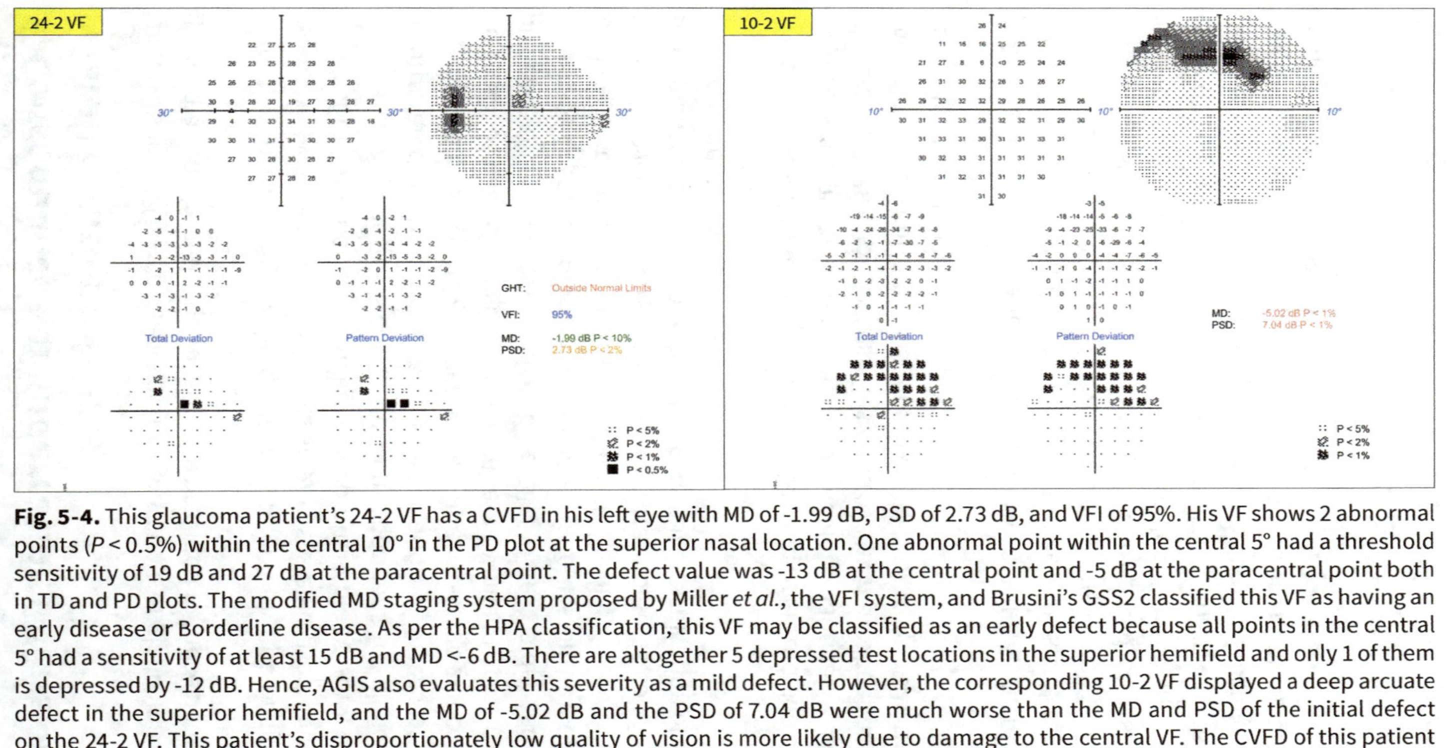

Fig. 5-4. This glaucoma patient's 24-2 VF has a CVFD in his left eye with MD of -1.99 dB, PSD of 2.73 dB, and VFI of 95%. His VF shows 2 abnormal points ($P < 0.5\%$) within the central 10° in the PD plot at the superior nasal location. One abnormal point within the central 5° had a threshold sensitivity of 19 dB and 27 dB at the paracentral point. The defect value was -13 dB at the central point and -5 dB at the paracentral point both in TD and PD plots. The modified MD staging system proposed by Miller *et al.*, the VFI system, and Brusini's GSS2 classified this VF as having an early disease or Borderline disease. As per the HPA classification, this VF may be classified as an early defect because all points in the central 5° had a sensitivity of at least 15 dB and MD <-6 dB. There are altogether 5 depressed test locations in the superior hemifield and only 1 of them is depressed by -12 dB. Hence, AGIS also evaluates this severity as a mild defect. However, the corresponding 10-2 VF displayed a deep arcuate defect in the superior hemifield, and the MD of -5.02 dB and the PSD of 7.04 dB were much worse than the MD and PSD of the initial defect on the 24-2 VF. This patient's disproportionately low quality of vision is more likely due to damage to the central VF. The CVFD of this patient was grossly underappreciated by the current glaucoma disease severity grading scale. However, only the 10-2 VF test with finer spacing in the central area could reveal and measure the severity of the central VF loss.

5. Consequences of underrating CVFDs on related health problems

Underrating CVFDs in patients at the early stage of glaucoma or suspected glaucoma can affect the quality of care provided to these patients.

In this discussion, early glaucoma refers to open-angle glaucoma associated with an MD ≤-6 dB. This staging system based on MD value is in contrast to the American Academy of Ophthalmology (AAO) and American Glaucoma Society (AGS) coding recommendations for glaucoma severity incorporated in the International Classification of Diseases, 10th Revision staging code.[13] AAO and AGC define mild or early-stage glaucoma as having no VF abnormalities present on any white-on-white VF test. In addition, the presence of a paracentral defect on a 10-2 VF test is defined as at least 3 contiguous depressed points along an arcuate-like pattern on the PD plot with at least 1 point depressed at the < 1% level or 2 points depressed at the < 2% level. A defect in 1 of the 4 central points is considered severe-stage glaucoma by AAO and the International Classification of Diseases, 10th Revision Codes.

Therefore, a definite controversy exists between the current glaucoma staging systems and the criteria of the International Classification of Diseases 10th Revision Codes. This controversy may affect not only billing and reimbursement but most importantly how frequently these patients are seen and tested in clinical practice.

A patient may have central VF damage on 10-2 VF and OCT imaging. That central damage may not be revealed by the 24-2 VF test. Based on 24-2 VF results that patient's disease severity often tends to be staged as without damage or with early damage (vide our represented case series). Consequently, such a patient may face difficulties. For instance, that patient may not be considered for treatment and followed up once a year or less. Patients may also be undertreated due to this wrong staging of the disease and the possibility of progression to blindness or visual impairment is substantially underestimated.

References

1. De Moraes CG, Sun A, Jarukasetphon R, Rajshekhar R, Shi L, Blumberg DM, Liebmann JM, Ritch R, Hood DC. Association of macular visual field measurements with glaucoma staging systems. JAMA Ophthalmol. 2019 Feb 1;137(2):139-145. https://doi.org/10.1001/jamaophthalmol.2018.5398

2. Hodapp E, Parrish II RK, Anderson DR. Clinical decisions in glaucoma. St Louis, MO: Mosby Co; 1993.

3. Susanna R Jr, Vessani RM. Staging glaucoma patient: why and how? Open Ophthalmol J. 2009;3:59-64. https://doi.org/10.2174/1874364100903020059

4. Brusini P, Filacorda S. Enhanced glaucoma staging system (GSS 2) for classifying functional damage in glaucoma. J Glaucoma. 2006;15(1):40-46. https://doi.org/10.1097/01.ijg.0000195932.48288.97

5. Mills RP, Budenz DL, Lee PP, et al. Categorizing the stage of glaucoma from pre-diagnosis to end-stage disease. Am J Ophthalmol. 2006;141:24-30. https://doi.org/10.1016/j.ajo.2005.07.044

6. The Field Analyzer Primer: Excellent Perimetry.

7. Aulhorn E, Karmeyer H. Frequency distribution in early glaucomatous visual field defects. Doc Ophthalmol Proc Series. 1977;14:75-83.

8. Advanced Glaucoma Intervention Study (AGIS). 2. Visual field test scoring and reliability. Ophthalmology. 1994;101:1445-55. https://doi.org/10.1016/S0161-6420(94)31171-7

9. Susanna R, Vessani R. ARVO E-Abstract 5287. Invest Ophthalmol Vis Sci. 2009;1:50.

10. Artes PH, Hutchison DM, Nicolela MT, LeBlanc RP, Chauhan BC. Threshold and variability properties of matrix frequency-doubling technology and standard automated perimetry in glaucoma. Invest Ophthalmol Vis Sci. 2005;46(7):2451-2457. https://doi.org/10.1167/iovs.05-0135

11. Abadia B, Ferreras A, Calvo P, Fogagnolo P, Figus M, Pajarin AB. Effect of the eye tracking system on the reproducibility of measurements obtained with spectral-domain optical coherence tomography in glaucoma. J Glaucoma. 2017;26(7):638-645. https://doi.org/10.1097/IJG.0000000000000690

12. Chakravarti T, Moghimi S, De Moraes CG, Weinreb RN. Central-most Visual Field Defects in Early Glaucoma. J Glaucoma. 2021 Mar 1;30(3):e68-e75. https://doi.org/10.1097/IJG.0000000000001747

13. Brämer GR. International statistical classification of diseases and related health problems. Tenth revision. World Health Stat Q. 1988;41(1):32-6.

Chapter 6

The utility of the 10-2 visual field test for the evaluation and management of central defects in early glaucoma

Chapter 6 weighs the utility of the 10-2 for the evaluation and management of central defects in early glaucoma. This chapter explains how and why a 10-2 VF test pattern would be a better instrument to recognize CVFDs or glaucomatous macular damage in the central 10°. This chapter also addresses whether the 10-2 VF test provides sufficient additional information to the 24-2 VF test to justify its routine use in clinical practice for the evaluation and management of early-stage glaucoma.

1. Advantage of the 10-2 test for identifying CVFDs

Detection of CVFDs increases when a test pattern with a spatial grain is finer than the typical 6° X 6° grid of the 24-2. By comparison, the 10-2 threshold VF test measures the central 10° with 68 points, more than 5 times the points measured in the central 10° by the 24-2 and 30-2 test patterns (Fig. 6-1). These points are all 2° apart, just 1° from either side of the horizontal and vertical meridians. As a result of this greater sensitivity, this test pattern can improve the detection of paracentral and central scotomas involving only a small area of the VF at or near fixation which may be missed with 24-2 and 30-2 perimetry.[1-7] Hence, the 10-2 test pattern identifies a greater number and more severe type of glaucomatous macular defects than a 24-2 test pattern as demonstrated by Figure 6-2. Figure 6-2 also provides evidence that 24-2 underestimates the severity of glaucomatous damage in the central 10°.

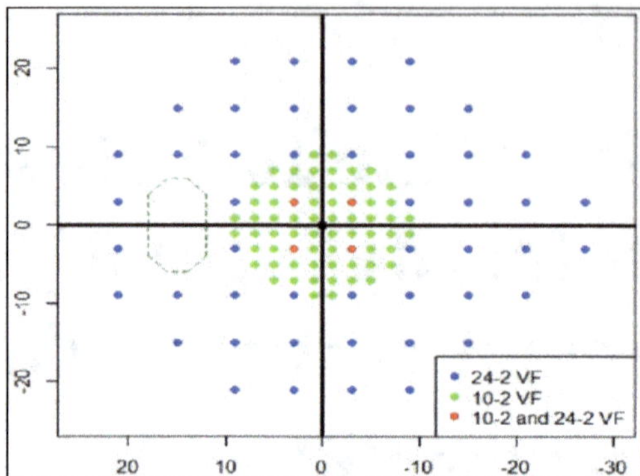

Fig. 6-1. Mapping of 10-2 and 24-2 VF test points. Blue and green circles represent test points in the 24-2 VF and 10-2 VF, respectively. Red circles show points tested by both the 24-2 and 10-2 VF. Reproduced from Asaoka.[8]

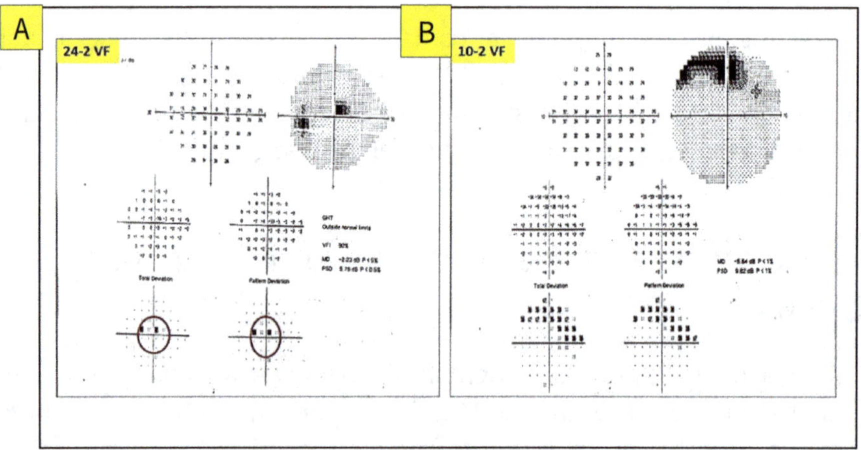

Fig. 6-2. IPFS on the 24-2 VF and corresponding dense PFS on the 10-2 test. **(A)** The VF of a patient recently diagnosed as a case of open-angle glaucoma. His 24-2 VF shows an IPFS in the superior hemifield within central 10° with 2 severely depressed abnormal test points P < 0.5%. One of those depressed test points is within the central 5°. His VFI value was reduced by 8% compared to the age-corrected normal value. The MD is -2.23 dB and the PSD is 5.78 dB. This CVFD is also evident on the greyscale of the 24-2 VF. **(B)** When this patient was tested on the same day with a 10-2 test pattern, this CVFD was more obvious as a superior dense arcuate-like PFS on a 10-2 VF with MD -5.64 dB and PSD 9.32 dB, much worse (severe) than the initial VF loss as detected on 24-2 VF.

2. Comparison of the diagnostic ability of the 24-2 and 10-2 strategies in the light of extant literature

Several studies have investigated how well the 24-2 and 10-2 VF tests correlate or agree with each other within the central 10°. The findings of these studies are important factors for determining the utility of 10-2 VF testing in early glaucoma. While some studies observed a distinct advantage of the 10-2 test pattern over the 24-2 for identifying CVFDs, some observed that the 10-2 test may not be essential for many patients. The second group demonstrated concurrence with each other (24-2 and 10-2) within the central 10° and suggested that the 24-2 VF test may be sufficient for detecting early central defects. We discuss both views.

3. Advantage of the 10-2 test pattern for identifying CVFDs

Traynis *et al.*[9] investigated the prevalence and characteristics of VF defects in the central 10° in glaucoma suspects and patients with mild glaucoma using a prospective design. They reported 53% abnormal 10-2 hemifields and 59% abnormal 24-2 hemifields. Of the eyes with normal 24-2 hemifields, 16% were classified as abnormal when the 10-2 test was used. Of the abnormal 10-2 hemifields, 68%, 8%, and 25% were arcuate-like, widespread, and other, respectively. Therefore, macular damage as seen on 10-2 VFs appears to occur almost as frequently as peripheral defects in patients with early glaucoma, and testing with the 24-2 VF alone can miss defects detected on the 10-2 VF. Park *et al.* compared the performance of 10-2 versus 24-2 VFs in detecting the progression of IPFS in glaucomatous eyes.[10] On evaluating the progression of CVFDs in glaucomatous eyes, they reported that eyes with greater progression were significantly detected in 10-2 than in 24-2 analyses (24 versus 11 eyes; $P = 0.007$). This difference became greater within the central 10° (24 versus 4 eyes; $P < 0.001$). These findings suggest that closer surveillance of the central VF using testing algorithms with closely spaced grids is necessary for eyes with IPFS.[10]

Ekici *et al.*[11] investigated the central VF defects among 4 phenotypes of glaucomatous optic discs in a cross-sectional study. Optic disc phenotypes were determined in eyes with definite or suspected glaucoma that had a 24–2 VF with MD <-12 dB and a 10–2 VF. 10–2 VFs were classified as abnormal based on CC. The study identified 4 glaucomatous optic disc phenotypes in 448 eyes of 309 patients: focal ischemic (*n* = 121), generalized cup enlargement (*n* = 109), myopic glaucoma (*n* = 66), and senile sclerotic (n = 152). The study observed that the severity and prevalence of central VF loss varied among different glaucomatous optic disc phenotypes. They concluded that eyes with focal ischemic and myopic glaucoma optic disc phenotypes are more likely to have 10-2 VF loss, particularly in early disease and may benefit especially from testing with both 10-2 and 24-2 VF tests.

4. 10-2 VF testing may be superfluous for many patients

4.1. Sullivan-Mee *et al.*

Sullivan-Mee *et al.*[4] investigated the clinical characteristics of 10-2 VF defects in patients diagnosed with glaucoma (mean MD <-6 dB on 24-2VF) or glaucoma suspects. They examined the 24-2 SITA Standard and 10-2 SITA Fast VF tests of 354 eyes with glaucoma, ocular hypertension, or glaucoma suspects. Of the 236 eyes with no defect on the 24-2 VF test, only 6.4% presented a defect on 10-2 VF. This study observed that the presence and severity of 10-2 VF loss could be generally estimated using results from 24-2 VF testing and spectral domain-OCT imaging and concluded that the information obtained by 10-2 VF testing may be superfluous for many patients.

4.2. Wu *et al.*

Wu *et al.*[12] compared the performance and diagnostic ability of the PSD values derived from the central 12 locations of the 24–2 VF test (C24–2) to the entire 10–2 test for detecting central VF abnormalities in eyes suspected of or at risk of having glaucoma. This study included 523 eyes with suspected glaucoma, or ocular hypertension, with 107 healthy control eyes. The sensitivities of the PSD values at 95% specificity were similar for early glaucoma cases with a 24-2 MD of -6 dB or better (10-2: 18.9%; Central-12: 17.9%; *P*=0.85, *n* = 515). Differentiating between early glaucoma and healthy eyes, the area under the receiver operating characteristic curve (AUROC) for the 10-2 PSD and 24-2 PSD was not significantly different ($P = 0.65$). This study showed that using PSD values, 10–2 and 24–2 tests identified central VF abnormalities in a similar number of eyes with suspected or at risk of having glaucoma.

4.3. West *et al.*

West *et al.*[13] compared the Central-12 and 10-2 TD and PD analyses at the < 5% and < 2% levels among 97 patients with early glaucoma with 65 normal control participants. The AUROC was not statistically different between the Central-12 and 10-2 VF tests for any of the 4 comparisons, ranging from 0.88 to 0.93 for the Central-12 tests and from 0.91 to 0.94 for the 10-2 tests.

4.4. Orbach *et al.*

The study by Orbach *et al.*[14] investigated whether glaucomatous central VF abnormalities can be more effectively detected using a qualitative, expert evaluation of the 10-2 test compared with the topographically correspond-ing central 12 locations of the 24-2 test (C24-2). No significant difference was observed in the sensitivity of detecting glaucoma cases at 95% specificity between the Central-12 and 10-2 VF. Similarly, no difference in sensitivity was found between the Central-12 and 10-2 tests using the PSD global index.

5. Defining a 10-2 VF defect in the light of published literature

The cluster rule is applied to identify abnormal hemifields on a 10-2 VF. A 10-2 VF defect is defined as a repeatable cluster of at least 3 contiguous abnormal points in the superior or inferior hemifield with at least 1 of the 3 points exceeding the 1% threshold or at least 2 of the points exceeding the 2% threshold.

Thus, a 10-2 VF is considered abnormal if the hemifield on the TD or PD plot is abnormal on 2 consecutive tests. Hemifields are classified as abnormal if there is a cluster of 3 or more contiguous points (5%, 5%, and 1% or 5%, 2%, and 2%) within a hemifield on either TD or PD plots.[9] Several studies have applied these criteria to both the TD and PD plots to define a 10-2 VF defect. However, some studies have used these criteria only in the PD plot to reduce false-positive results related to diffuse VF loss from non-glaucomatous etiologies.

6. Types and patterns of PFS on 10-2 VF

Both CC and types of pattern defects are used to identify and classify the 10-2 VF defects or PFS on 10-2. 10-2 VF defects are classified into different categories based on the pattern or shape of abnormal points in the hemifields. The CC are already mentioned above when defining 10-2 VF defects. Different types of pattern defects are described below.

Early glaucomatous macular damage is primarily arcuate-like RNFL damage. Configuration of arcuate-like damage on 10-2 should follow the characteristics of classic glaucomatous arcuate field defects on 24-2 VF. Arcuate VF defects are defined based on the appearance of the abnormal test point locations on the 10-2 test. To be classified as typical glaucomatous arcuate field defects on the 10-2, the abnormal region must follow an arc, stretching from the midline in the nasal field to the edge of the temporal field, and must be closer to fixation nasally than temporally.[6] Figure 6-3 shows examples of arcuate defects on the 10-2 VF. Some investigators have used simpler definitions for classifying arcuate-like defects. As per their definition, if repeatable cluster points are present on both sides of the vertical hemifield midline, the pattern is considered an arcuate defect.[4]

6.1. Classifying PFS on 10-2 VF

The basic definition of an arcuate parafoveal scotoma on the 10-2 VF test has been further modified by researchers to explain its characteristics and severity both quantitatively and qualitatively.[4,9,15,16]

6.1.1. Median central arcuate scotoma

The term "median central arcuate" was first introduced for a special type of arcuate defect on 10-2 VF (Fig. 6-4).[6] To elucidate median central arcuate on 10-2 VF, Hood *et al.*[6] applied the relationship between RNFL damage and VF defects.

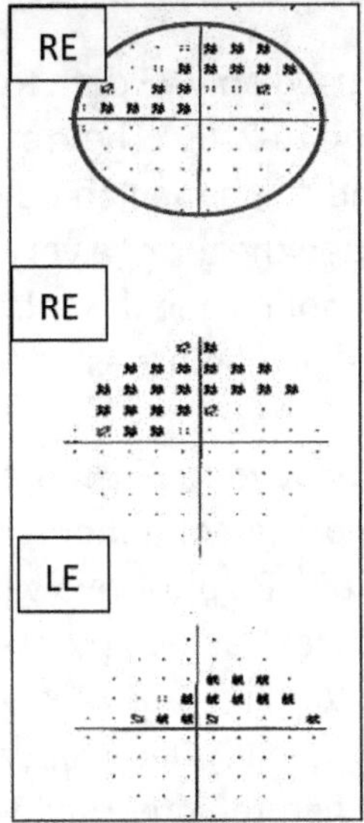

Fig. 6-3. Examples of complete arcuate defects on the 10-2 test. Reproduced from Hood *et al.*[6]

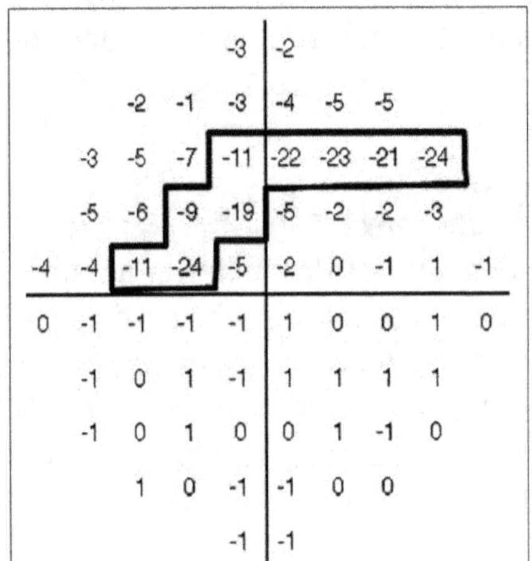

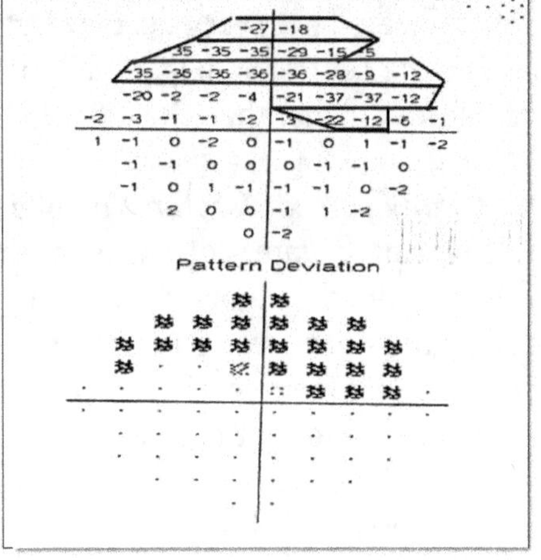

Fig. 6-4. Typical or median central arcuate defect. **(Left)** PFS on 10-2 VF described as a median central arcuate defect. Reproduced from Hood *et al.*[6] The region within the black borders includes the abnormal points with a median deviation ≤ -9 dB. **(Right)** PFS consisting of abnormal 10-2 test points **(black borders)** with "very deep defect". The sensitivity loss range is -12 dB to -35 dB at abnormal test point locations.

However, some clinicians used only VF data to explain the characteristics of "median central arcuate" on 10-2 VF.[16] They revised and modified the term "median central arcuate" and "high median defect depth". Instead of high median defect depth, they used the term "a very deep defect" (-12 dB to -35 dB) at abnormal 10-2 VF test points and described an arcuate defect with a very deep defect at abnormal test points as a "deep arcuate scotoma".[15,16]

6.1.2. Deep arcuate scotoma or advanced arcuate defect

This type of arcuate scotoma is a continuous, dense, superior or inferior hemifield defect ($P < 1\%$ on TD or PD plot) involving both nasal and temporal quadrants with very deep defect at test points and involving the central 5° from the fixation of 10-2 VF (Fig. 6-5A). Deep arcuate defects occur in and near the foveal region of the VF. Deep arcuate scotomas show greater (worse) MD and PSD values than the other milder types of arcuate defects on the 10-2 VF test.

6.1.3. Shallow arcuate scotoma or moderate arcuate defect

The shallow arcuate scotoma is similar to a deep arcuate scotoma except not associated with very deep defect at abnormal test points and does not involve the central 5°. (Fig. 6-5B). In this defect type, 10-2 MD and PSD are moderately higher than the other milder types of arcuate defects.

6.1.4. Partial arcuate scotoma or mild arcuate defect

This type of arcuate scotoma is continuous but less dense (fewer abnormal points) than a shallow arcuate scotoma, superior or inferior hemifield defect, does not involve the central 5° of 10-2 VF fixation, and may include both nasal and temporal quadrants. The partial arcuate scotoma (Fig. 6-5C) is milder in severity than the shallow arcuate scotoma. In this defect type, MD and PSD values are lower (better) than the other 2 types of arcuate defects described above.

6.1.5. Nasal defect or incomplete arcuate scotoma

In nasal defects (incomplete arcuate), the abnormal points are restricted largely to the nasal field (Fig. 6-5D). Another definition of "incomplete arcuate" is when abnormal points are largely scattered in the nasal field. Some classification systems evaluate this pattern of 10-2 defects with the following definition:[4] if all abnormal, repeatable cluster points are limited to 1 quadrant, the pattern is considered a nasal defect.

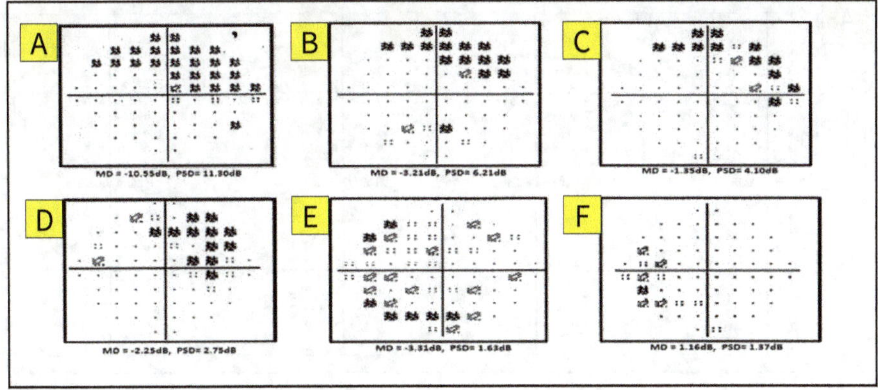

Fig. 6-5. Types and patterns of PFS on 10-2 VF. **(A)** Deep arcuate scotoma or advanced arcuate defect. **(B)** Shallow arcuate scotoma or moderate arcuate defect. **(C)** Partial arcuate scotoma or mild arcuate defect. **(D)** Nasal defect. **(E)** Widespread defect. **(F)** Cluster defect.

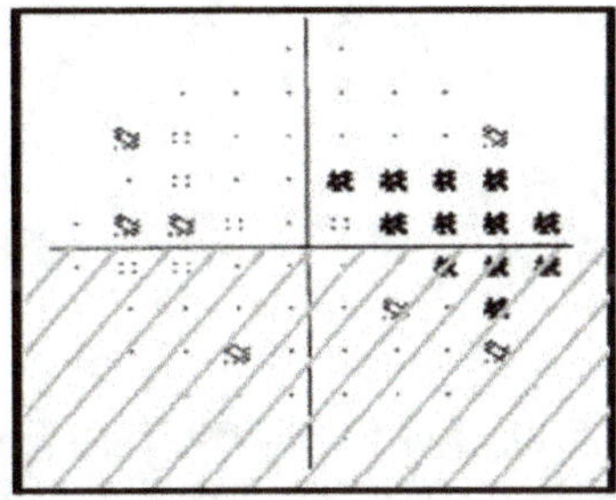

Fig. 6-6. Other defects or temporal defects. Reproduced from Traynis *et al.*[9]

6.1.6. Widespread defect

The widespread category is defined as a loss in all 4 quadrants on both TD and PD plots that do not appear as arcuate-like defects (Fig. 6-5E).

6.1.7. Other defect or temporal defect

Abnormal hemifields that do not fall into either of these categories are classified as other. They are predominately scattered abnormal test points across the field or predominately located in the temporal quadrants (Fig. 6-6).

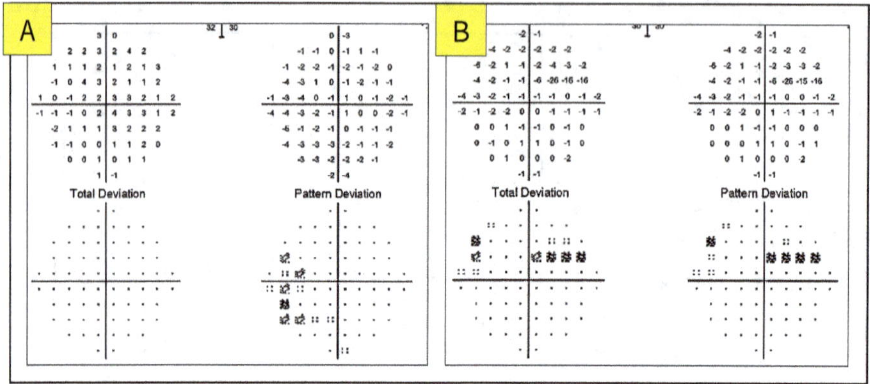

Fig. 6-7. Examples of cluster defects on a 10-2 VF test of 2 different patients. **(A)** In the right eye, a cluster is formed by abnormal points with *P* < 2%, 2%, and 5%. Very shallow defects are seen at the 10-2 test points as shown in the PD numerical plots; MD and PSD values are also very low (MD = -1.16 dB, PSD = 1.37 dB), indicating minor defects. **(B)** A cluster is formed (in the patient's right eye) on 10-2 VF by abnormal points *P* < 1%, with high defects such as -26dB, -15 dB, -16 dB at abnormal test points. As expected, the MD is -2.00 dB and PSD 4.18 dB on this VF, greater (worse) than the MD and PSD value of the VF in *(A)*.

6.1.8. Cluster defect

A cluster is defined as 3 contiguous abnormal points with *P* < 5%, 5%, and 1% or *P* < 5%, 2%, and 2% depressed from the normative database, within a hemifield on either TD or PD plot (Fig. 6-5F). Figure 6-7 presents examples of cluster defects of 2 different patients on a 10-2 VF test with varying disease severity. Though both VFs (Figure 6-7A and Figure 6-7B) are examples of cluster defects on the 10-2 VF test, the clinical importance of these 2 cluster defects is different. Glaucomatous defects are thought to progress from small, shallow deficits to large, deep defects. Disease severity is higher in the eye with the type of cluster defects shown in Figure 6-7B than in Figure 6-7A. Hence, the patient with cluster defect depicted in Figure 6-7B should be closely monitored.

7. The role of 10-2 VF for detecting and monitoring the progression of CVFDs

VF progression occurs either by intensification or enlargement of an existing scotoma or by a combination of these 2 processes. The VF progression rate is likely to be greater in the central 10° area and could directly threaten patients' visual function compared to glaucomatous damage involving the 10°–30° region. Therefore, it is important to investigate the pattern of VF progression within the central 10° region.

It is easier to detect VF progression in the central field with steeper slopes of VF sensitivity than in the periphery because the central test points have lower test-retest variability than the peripheral points. Further, central VF progression is related to vascular risk factors, and OCT angiography demonstrates that central VF involvement has been reported to be associated with vessel density loss.[17]

For detecting and monitoring VF progression within the central 10° of fixation, the performance of 10-2 VF is better in eyes with IPFS on 24-2 VF.[10,18] The superior performance of the 10-2 test compared with the 24-2 test is likely the result of the greater number and even distribution of condensed test points in a closely spaced grid within the tested area. While the 10-2 VF test comprises 68 test locations, conventional 24-2 perimetry comprises only 12 test locations for evaluating the central 10°. Conventional perimetry lacks detailed spatial information due to its rectangular test point arrangement with a spacing of 6° X 6° that omits the 6° central VF region. Local enhancement of test point condensation will help early detection and exact demarcation of the pattern of the scotoma. Further, it will provide the information to detect progression earlier than can be detected with conventional perimetric grids.[19]

8. The role of 10-2 VF tests in different stages of glaucoma

Tomairek *et al.* evaluated the role of the 10-2 VF test in different stages of glaucoma.[20] In early glaucoma, evaluating eyes with CVFD by 10-2 VF test and OCT would be a beneficial addition to the 24-2 test for precise diagnosis and proper management. Glaucomatous eyes with CVFD or macular involvement may require reclassification to severe glaucoma after evaluation with more competent tools. These supplementary investigations with the 10-2 testing may provide a more realistic representation of the true extent of VF loss that reflects the actual severity of the disease and aids in accurately staging the disease severity.

Although the role of the 10-2 test is not as crucial in moderate and severe glaucoma as it is in early cases, it is still useful for the assessment of residual central visual function in severe cases with absolute central 10° defects on the 24-2 test for precise management. In advanced loss, following up glaucoma patients with 10-2 VFs is especially advantageous when the central points on 24-2 VF are affected. A better understanding of patterns of CVFDs and their development over time is of great significance in improving the management of advanced glaucoma, for which the 10-2 test is essential.

9. Baseline 10-2 VF defects: an effective predictor of subsequent 24-2 VF progression

A longitudinal study recently identified that baseline 10-2 VF loss has greater specificity and precision for predicting subsequent worsening of 24-2 glaucomatous VF loss.[21] They studied patients diagnosed with POAG and glaucoma suspects. Eligibility required 2 good-quality baseline 10-2 VF tests followed by a minimum of 5 good quality 24-2 VF tests over a period of at least 3 years. They observed that in early glaucoma, the 10-2 VF test has a definite predictive value even when the central points of the 24-2 VF are normal. In POAG patients, eyes with a baseline 10-2 VF defect may have a 4-times greater rate of 24-2 MD deterioration compared with eyes with no 10-2 VF defect at baseline. In contrast, eyes with abnormal baseline central 24-2 points have only a 3-times greater rate of 24-2 MD progression compared with eyes with no abnormal baseline central 24-2 points.[21]

10. Suggestion for implementing the 10-2 VFs to a baseline protocol

Sullivan-Mee *et al.*[21] observed that baseline 10-2 VF defect is the most effective predictor of subsequent 24-2 VF progression. The primary result of this study is that the presence/absence of baseline 10-2 VF loss can provide insight regarding the future course of glaucomatous disease. Therefore, implementing a 10-2 VF test as a baseline protocol may improve baseline decisions regarding the degree of treatment and surveillance intensity. Again, in a separate study, Wu *et al.*[18] compared 10-2 and 24-2 VF to detect progressive central VF loss in glaucoma eyes with early central abnormalities. They observed that global trend-based analysis with the 10-2 MD values detected central VF progression earlier than C24-2 MD values in eyes with early CVFD when the specificities of the two methods were matched. Together, these findings suggest the inference that the 10-2 VF test may provide unique predictive value in early glaucoma for enhancing baseline clinical risk assessment even when the central points of the 24-2 VF are normal.

POAG is generally a bilateral disorder and is often asymmetric, particularly in the early stages. Hence, there may be a possibility that the fellow eye can be in the pre-perimetric stage. For glaucoma patients with one eye with glaucomatous damage and the other being a suspect, a baseline 10-2 VF test may be helpful for early detection and monitoring of glaucoma, specifically in such fellow eyes which are normal on the 24-2 VF test. Additionally, there are other clinical advantages of baseline 10-2 VF testing for assessing risk analysis in eyes exhibiting disc hemorrhage. Such eyes demonstrate faster VF progression on 10-2 versus 24-2 VF tests. Thereby, a baseline 10-2 VF test could guide initial treatment intensity. Consequently, clinicians may consider changing glaucoma practice by implementing the 10-2 VFs to a baseline protocol to serve patients better, rather than keep waiting for additional evidence to develop.

11. Retinal nerve fiber layer optical texture analysis (ROTA) and 10-2 VF assessment in glaucoma

Contrary to the belief that the fovea and macula are not affected until the late stages of glaucoma, papillofoveal and papillomacular bundle defects as well as associated central VF defects at the corresponding VF test locations are common in early glaucoma. A reliable method for detecting functional and structural deficits over the macula in glaucoma is to examine RNFL defects in the papillomacular and papillofoveal bundles. RNFL optical texture analysis (ROTA), a new algorithm, can reveal the path of the axonal fiber bundles over a wide field by exhibiting the optical texture of axonal fiber bundles embedded in OCT scans.[22] In addition to the arcuate bundles, ROTA distinctively reveals the route of papillomacular and papillofoveal bundles, which are difficult to recognize from red-free photographs because the visibility of the RNFL drops with age.[23] Other reasons for poor visibility of papillomacular and papillofoveal bundles in red-free photographs are hypopigmented fundus, media opacities, and diffuse RNFL thinning.[23] They are barely visible in conventional OCT analysis.

The ROTA algorithm can precisely define the location and extent of RNFL defects within and beyond the macula. The arcuate bundle represents the axonal fiber bundle spreading along the superior and inferior temporal retinal vascular arcades outside the macula (18° or approximately 5.5 mm; Fig. 6-8A). The papillomacular bundle corresponds to the axonal fiber bundles projected from the macula (Fig. 6-8B), except for those projected from the fovea (5°, or approximately 1.5 mm), which are labelled as the papillofoveal bundle (Fig. 6-8C). The papillofoveal bundle is further classified into:

1. The arcuate papillofoveal bundle, which includes axonal fiber bundles projected from the temporal fovea arching over the foveola to the optic disc (Fig. 6-8D).
2. The horizontal papillofoveal bundle, which comprises axonal fiber bundles running mostly parallel to the foveola-Bruch's membrane opening center axis from the nasal fovea to the optic disc (Fig. 6-8E).

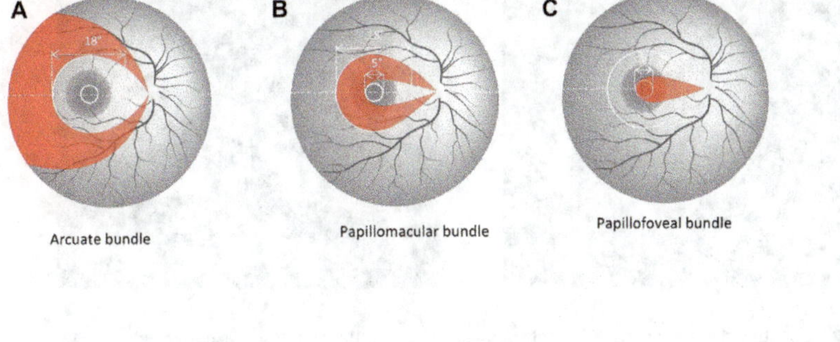

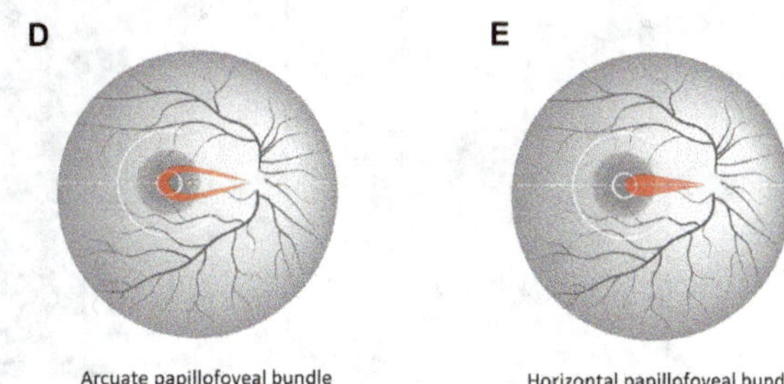

Fig. 6-8. Types of axonal fiber bundles classified by their origins in the retina. **(A)** The arcuate bundle arises outside the macula (18°, or approximately 5.5 mm) along the superior and inferior temporal vascular arcades. **(B)** The papillomacular bundle contains axonal fiber bundles projected from the macula, except those projected from the fovea (5°, or approximately 1.5 mm). **(C)** The papillofoveal bundle includes axonal fiber bundles projected from the fovea. The papillofoveal bundle is further classified into **(D)** the arcuate papillofoveal bundle, which consists of axonal fiber bundles projected from the temporal fovea arching over the foveola to the optic disc, and **(E)** the horizontal papillofoveal bundle, which contains axonal fiber bundles running mostly parallel to each other from the nasal fovea to the optic disc. Figure and legend reproduced from Leung *et al.*[22]

It is also possible to map individual VF stimulus projections topographically on the ROTA map to explain the location-by-location structure-function association (Fig. 6-9).

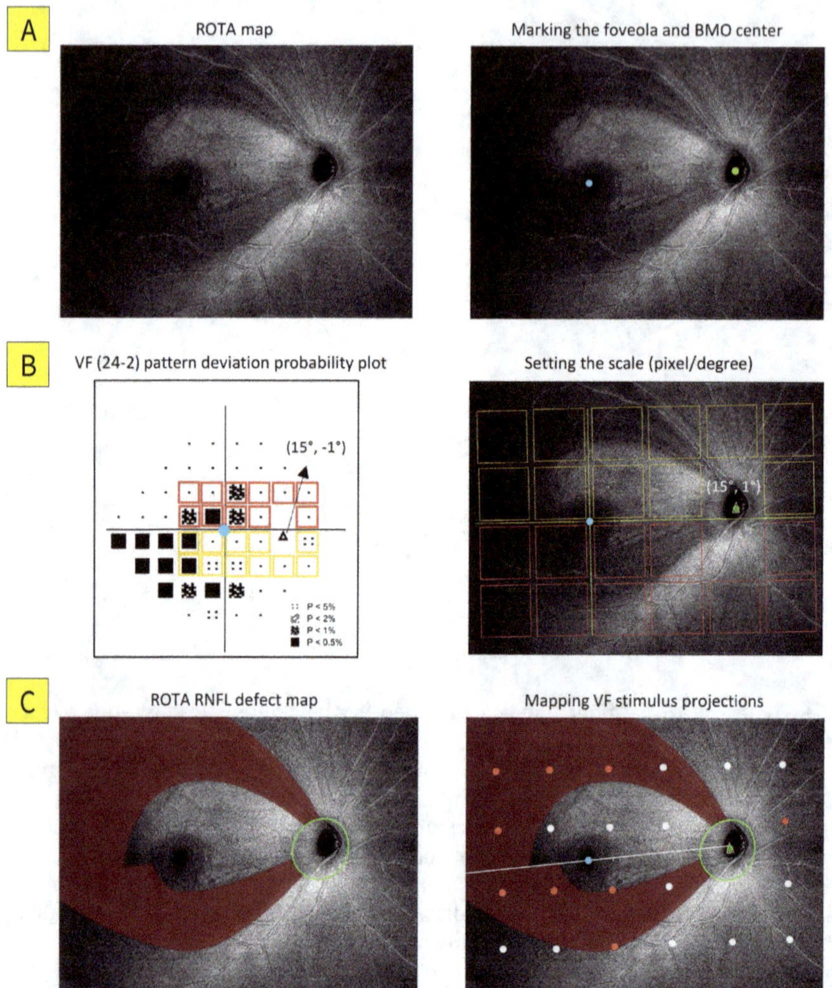

Fig. 6-9. Mapping of VF stimulus projections onto the RNFL ROTA map. **(A)** Bruch's membrane opening (BMO) center **(green dot)** and the foveola **(blue dot)** are marked on the ROTA map. **(B)** Alignments of the center of the blind spot (indicated by a triangle in the PD plot) (15°, -1°) relative to the central fixation (0, 0) **(left panel)** were exported from the HFA and transposed onto the BMO center and foveola of the ROTA map, respectively, to set the scale (pixels per degree) for mapping the VF stimulus projections onto the ROTA map **(right panel). (C)** Individual VF stimulus projections, 0.43 in size (Goldmann size III) and spaced 6° apart, in the superior hemifield are mapped to the inferior hemiretina and vice versa. Red dots on the ROTA map represent locations with a VF pattern deviation probability value of < 5%; white dots represent locations with a VF PD probability value of > 5%. Figure and legend reproduced from Leung *et al.*[22]

11.1 The role of the 10-2 VF test to detect VF loss associated with papillomacular and papillofoveal bundle defects

A recent study applied ROTA in 204 eyes with early glaucoma from 171 patients to investigate:

1. What were the most common patterns of RNFL defects in early glaucoma.
2. How often the papillomacular and papillofoveal bundles were involved.
3. How likely was a VF stimulus projected onto a papillomacular or papillofoveal bundle defect to show an abnormal sensitivity.[24]

Of the 204 eyes, 71.6% and 17.2% demonstrated papillomacular and papillofoveal bundle defects, respectively; only 25% of eyes showed isolated arcuate bundle defects without involvement of papillomacular or papillofoveal bundles.[24] However, the remaining 75.0% demonstrated varying degrees of papillomacular bundle or papillofoveal bundle loss. The pattern of RNFL defects varied, with the most common being concomitant involvement of the inferior arcuate bundle and the inferior papillomacular bundle (20.6%).[24] The high percentage of eyes with inferior papillomacular bundle defects is indicative of and consistent with the IVZ in the RNFL thickness and GICPL thickness probability maps described by Hood[25] and Hood et al.[26] in Chapter 3. Adding to their finding, the present study highlights the unanticipated involvement of the papillofoveal bundle in early glaucoma, which otherwise would not be visible with conventional OCT RNFL and GCIPL thickness analysis. Again, conserving the papillofoveal and papillomacular bundles is essential in the management of glaucoma patients. More rigorous monitoring and treatment regimens would be indicated in patients with papillomacular bundle defects, and more so with papillofoveal bundle defects, due to the higher risk of central vision loss and development of visual disability.

It was observed that only eyes with arcuate bundle defects, but not those with papillofoveal and papillomacular bundle defects, were associated with VF defects in the corresponding hemifield on the 24-2 VF test. The structure-function discordance is recognized because only 4 test locations of the 24-2 VF test points correspond to the macula (18°). However, VF defects associated with papillomacular or papillofoveal bundle defects could be detected in the 24-2 test when concomitant involvement of the arcuate bundle was present. The structure-function association analysis by hemifields supports the ability of ROTA in distinguishing arcuate bundle defects versus papillomacular and papillofoveal bundle defects. Figure 6-10 illustrates the 4 central 24-2 VF test locations and RNFL bundle defects on RNFL ROTA maps that were used to determine the likelihood of 10-2 VF sensitivity abnormality. Except for those 4 central 24-2 VF test points, other 24-2 VF stimulus projections extend beyond the central 18°. The present study highlights the importance of applying VF tests with a higher sampling density over the central 18°, such as the 10-2 test and the 24-2C test,[1] to detect VF loss associated with papillomacular and papillofoveal bundle defects. Further, this study alerts against the labelling of pre-perimetric glaucoma without considering the spatial correspondence between VF stimulus projections and RNFL defects.

11.2. The role of ROTA in enhancing the understanding and prediction of 10-2 VF abnormalities

Another study also observed a strong association between ROTA RNFL bundle defects and VF abnormalities at corresponding topographic test locations on both the 24-2 and 10-2 maps.[27] Pointwise analyses of the PD/TD plots further validated that papillomacular and papillofoveal bundle defects closely corresponded to central VF loss at the 10-2 test locations. The individual PD/TD plots showed ROTA's precise representation of preserved and damaged areas of the 10-2 VF, which were not always evident on the 24-2 map due to lower test location density. This finding can be attributed to the 10- 2 VF map's representation of each quadrant (17 test locations) by only 1 central test location on the 24-2 VF map. This low density of test locations leads to a potential loss of detecting central VF damage details on a 24-2 VF map.

The inclusion of structural information from ROTA RNFL bundle defects significantly improves the detection of 10-2 VF abnormalities at specific test points. This research specifies the pointwise odds ratio for the association between the presence of RNFL bundle defect and the likelihood of abnormality ($P < 0.05$) at individual 10-2 test locations (Fig. 6-11).[27]

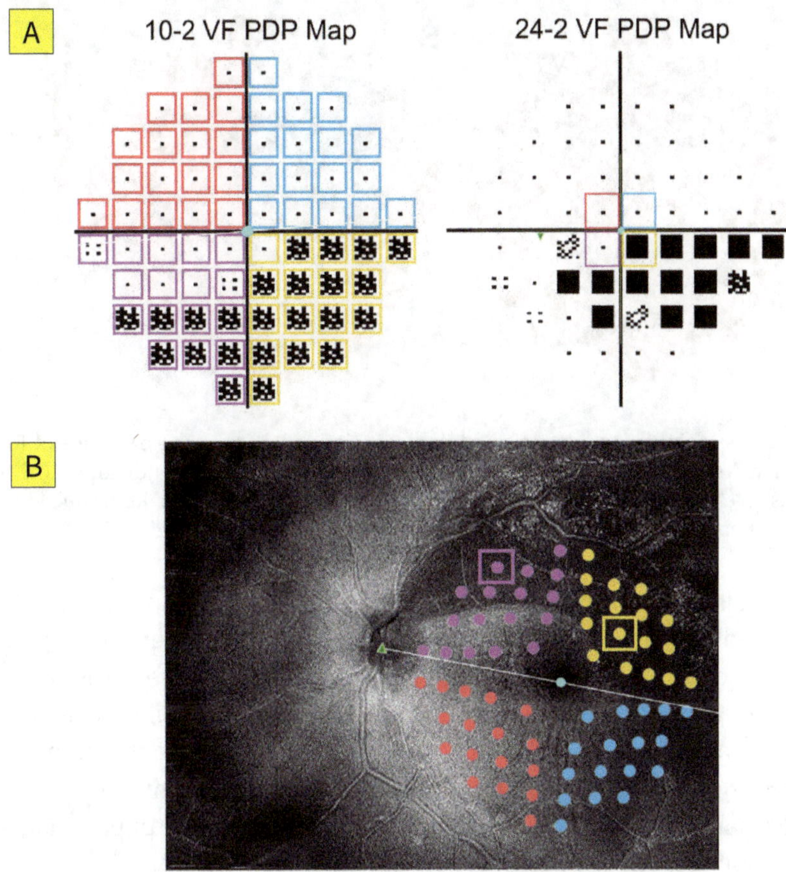

Fig. 6-10. Illustration of the central four 24-2 VF test locations and RNFL bundle defects on ROTA maps that are used to determine the likelihood of 10-2 VF sensitivity abnormality. **(A)** represents the 10-2 VF PD probability (PDP) map divided by 4 quadrants **(left panel)** and the related 4 central 24-2 test locations **(right panel)**. **(B)** The 10-2 VF stimulus projections superimposed on the related regions on the ROTA map. Both 10-2 test locations, indicated by purple and yellow squares, exhibit abnormalities on the 10-2 PDP map (*P* < 1%) and project over an RNFL bundle defect. However, while the central 24-2 test location corresponding to the yellow test point displays an abnormality (*P* < 0.5%), the central 24-2 test location corresponding to the purple test point remains within normal limits. Figure and legend reproduced from Kamalipour *et al.*[27]

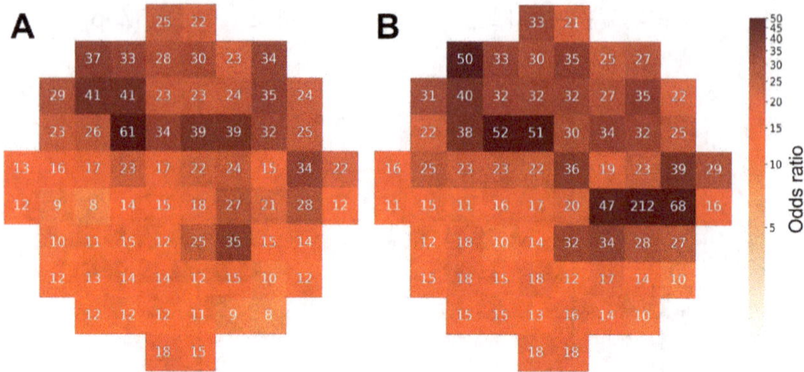

Fig. 6-11. The pointwise odds ratios for the association between the presence of RNFL bundle defects on ROTA and the likelihood of abnormality ($P < 5\%$) at individual 10-2 test locations on **(A)** PD probability and **(B)** TD probability (right eye format). Reproduced from Kamalipour *et al.*[27]

The findings of the present study highlight the important role of ROTA RNFL bundle defect assessment in enhancing the understanding and prediction of 10-2 VF abnormalities at a more refined level. It is evident that a strong topographic concordance exists between papillomacular and papillofoveal RNFL bundle defects on ROTA and central defects on the 10-2 VF test. Hence, the authors of the study recommend performing 10-2 VF test in early glaucoma when ROTA demonstrates evidence of papillomacular and/or papillofoveal RNFL bundle involvement.

References

1. De Moraes CG, Hood DC, Thenappan A, et al. 24-2 visual fields miss central defects shown on 10-2 tests in glaucoma suspects, ocular hypertensives, and early glaucoma. Ophthalmology. 2017;124(10):1449-1456. https://doi.org/10.1016/j.ophtha.2017.04.021

2. Grillo LM, Wang DL, Ramachandran R, et al. The 24-2 visual field test misses central macular damage confirmed by the 10-2 visual field test and optical coherence tomography. Transl Vis Sci Technol. 2016;5(2):15. https://doi.org/10.1167/tvst.5.2.15

3. Park HY, Hwang BE, Shin HY, Park CK. Clinical clues to predict the presence of parafoveal scotoma on Humphrey 10-2 visual field using a Humphrey 24-2 visual field. Am J Ophthalmol. 2016;161:150-159. https://doi.org/10.1016/j.ajo.2015.10.007

4. Sullivan-Mee M, Tran MT, Pensyl D, Tsan G, Katiyar S. Prevalence, features, and severity of glaucomatous visual field loss measured with the 10-2 achromatic threshold visual field test. Am J Ophthalmol. 2016;168:40-51. https://doi.org/10.1016/j.ajo.2016.05.003

5. Hood DC, Raza AS, de Moraes CG, Liebmann JM, Ritch R. Glaucomatous damage of the macula. Prog Retin Eye Res. 2013;32:1-21. https://doi.org/10.1016/j.preteyeres.2012.08.003

6. Hood DC, Raza AS, de Moraes CG, et al. Initial arcuate defects within the central 10 degrees in glaucoma. Invest Ophthalmol Vis Sci. 2011;52(2):940-946. https://doi.org/10.1167/iovs.10-5803

7. Langerhorst CT, Carenini LL, Bakker D, De Bie-Raakman MAC. Measurements for description of very early glaucomatous field defects: perimetry update. New York, NY: Kugler Publications; 1997:67-73.

8. Asaoka R. Measuring visual field progression in the central 10 degrees using additional information from central 24 degrees visual fields and 'lasso regression'. PLoS One. 2013;8(8). https://doi.org/10.1371/journal.pone.0072199

9. Traynis I, De Moraes CG, Raza AS, Liebmann JM, Ritch R, Hood DC. Prevalence and nature of early glaucomatous defects in the central 10° of the visual field. JAMA Ophthalmol. 2014;132(3):291-297. https://doi.org/10.1001/jamaophthalmol.2013.7656

10. Park SC, Kung Y, Su D, Simonson JL, Furlanetto RL, Liebmann JM, Ritch R. Parafoveal scotoma progression in glaucoma: Humphrey 10-2 versus 24-2 visual field analysis. Ophthalmology. 2013;120(8):1546-1550. https://doi.org/10.1016/j.ophtha.2013.01.045

11. Ekici E, Moghimi S, Hou H, et al. Central visual field defects in patients with distinct glaucomatous optic disc phenotypes. Am J Ophthalmol. 2021;223:229-240. https://doi.org/10.1016/j.ajo.2020.10.015

12. Wu Z, Medeiros FA, Weinreb RN, Zangwill LM. Performance of the 10-2 and 24-2 visual field tests for detecting central visual field abnormalities in glaucoma. Am J Ophthalmol. 2018;196:10-17. https://doi.org/10.1016/j.ajo.2018.08.010

13. West ME, Sharpe GP, Hutchison DM, et al. Value of 10-2 visual field testing in glaucoma patients with early 24-2 visual field loss. Ophthalmology. 2021;128(4):545-553. https://doi.org/10.1016/j.ophtha.2020.08.033

14. Orbach A, Ang GS, Camp AS, et al. Qualitative evaluation of the 10-2 and 24-2 visual field tests for detecting central visual field abnormalities in glaucoma. Am J Ophthalmol. 2021;229:26-33. https://doi.org/10.1016/j.ajo.2021.02.015

15. Chakravarti T, Moghimi S, Weinreb RN. Prediction of central visual field severity in glaucoma. J Glaucoma. 2022;31(6):430-437. https://doi.org/10.1097/IJG.0000000000002031

16. Chakravarti T, Moghimi S, De Moraes CG, Weinreb RN. Central-most visual field defects in early glaucoma. J Glaucoma. 2021;30(3). https://doi.org/10.1097/IJG.0000000000001747

17. Kim EK, Park HY, Hong KE, et al. Investigation of progression pattern and associated risk factors in glaucoma patients with initial paracentral scotomas using Humphrey 10-2. Sci Rep. 2021;11:18609. https://doi.org/10.1038/s41598-021-97446-6

18. Wu Z, Medeiros FA, Weinreb RN, Girkin CA, Zangwill LM. Comparing 10-2 and 24-2 visual fields for detecting progressive central visual loss in glaucoma eyes with early central abnormalities. Ophthalmol Glaucoma. 2019;2(2):95-102. https://doi.org/10.1016/j.ogla.2019.01.003

19. Schiefer U, Papageorgiou E, Sample PA, et al. Spatial pattern of glaucomatous visual field loss obtained with regionally condensed stimulus arrangements. Invest Ophthalmol Vis Sci. 2010;51(11):5685-5689. https://doi.org/10.1167/iovs.09-5067

20. Tomairek RH, Aboud SA, Hassan M, Mohamed AH. Studying the role of 10-2 visual field test in different stages of glaucoma. Eur J Ophthalmol. 2020;30(4):706-713. https://doi.org/10.1177/1120672119836904

21. Sullivan-Mee M, Kimura B, Kee H, et al. Baseline 10-2 visual field loss as a predictor for future glaucoma progression. J Glaucoma. 2023;32(1):1-8. https://doi.org/10.1097/IJG.0000000000002138

22. Leung CK, Lam AKN, Weinreb RN, et al. Diagnostic assessment of glaucoma and non-glaucomatous optic neuropathy via retinal nerve fiber layer optical texture analysis. Nat Biomed Eng. 2022;6(5):593e604. https://doi.org/10.1038/ s41551-021-00813-x.

23. Sommer A, Quigley HA, Robin AL, Miller NR, Katz J, Arkell S. Evaluation of Nerve Fiber Layer Assessment. Arch Ophthalmol. 1984;102 (12): 1766-1771. https://doi.org/10.1001/archopht.1984.01040031430017

24. Leung CKS, Guo PY, Lam AKN. Retinal Nerve Fiber Layer Optical Texture Analysis: Involvement of the Papillomacular Bundle and Papillofoveal Bundle in Early Glaucoma. Ophthalmology. 2022 Sep;129(9):1043-1055. https://doi.org/10.1016/j.ophtha.2022.04.012

25. Hood DC. Improving our understanding, and detection, of glaucomatous damage: An approach based upon optical coherence tomography (OCT). Prog Retin Eye Res. 2017 Mar;57:46-75. https://doi.org/10.1016/j.preteyeres.2016.12.002

26. Hood DC, Raza AS, de Moraes CG, Johnson CA, Liebmann JM, Ritch R. The nature of macular damage in glaucoma as revealed by averaging optical coherence tomography data. Transl Vis Sci Technol. 2012 May 25;1(1):3. https://doi.org/10.1167/tvst.1.1.3

27. Kamalipour A, Moghimi S, Khosravi P, Tansuebchueasai N, Vasile C, Adelpour M, Gunasegaran G, Nishida T, Zangwill LM, Lam AKN, Leung CKS, Weinreb RN. Retinal Nerve Fiber Layer Optical Texture Analysis and 10-2 Visual Field Assessment in Glaucoma. Am J Ophthalmol. 2024 Oct;266:118-134. https://doi.org/10.1016/j.ajo.2024.05.013

Chapter 7

Prediction of 10-2 defects by central 24-2 defects

This chapter explains factors related to abnormal 24-2 VF points responsible for the presence of parafoveal scotomas on the 10-2 VF. It also elucidates how the characteristics and severity of PFS on the 10-2 VF could be anticipated by measuring the threshold sensitivity and the magnitude of sensitivity loss (defect value) at abnormal VF points in the central 12 points on a 24-2 VF in early glaucoma.[1] Early glaucoma is defined by an MD ≤ -6 dB on the 24-2 VF test.

1. Prediction of 10-2 defects by central 24-2 defects

Some studies have found that central defects on the 24-2 VF test can predict defects on the 10-2 VF test and that the severity of 10-2 VF loss is reasonably predictable based on the findings of the 24-2 VF test alone.[1-3] These predictions may offer 2 possible alternatives: conditions optimal for a 10-2 test or a 10-2 test may be redundant in early glaucoma with central defects.

In this section, we first present an overview of published literature that indicated prediction of the characteristics and severity of 10-2 VF loss, based on the findings of the 24-2 VF test. We then continue by highlighting the factors that determine the occurrence of PFS on the 10-2 test. Finally, we enlist the factors that influence the characteristics and severity of PFS on the 10-2 test.

2. Published literature predicting the severity of 10-2 VF loss based on findings of the 24-2 VF test

Park *et al.* examined factors related to the presence of PFS on Humphrey 10-2 VF in early glaucoma patients.[4] This study observed that the presence of abnormal 24-2 VF points $P < 0.5\%$ was significantly different between eyes with and without PFS on 10-2 VF ($P < 0.01$). Park *et al.* recommend that glaucomatous eyes with any central abnormal 24-2 VF points ($P < 0.5\%$ or $< 5\%$), correlating to mGCIPL thinning deserves attention, requiring a further evaluation with a 10-2VF test.[4]

Chakravarti *et al.* also evaluated the ability of the abnormal central-most 4 points and paracentral 8 points of the 24-2 VF test in predicting the severity of defects in the 10-2 test.[1] This research has added a novel and significant contribution to the field of central defects in early glaucoma because it indicated how to evaluate the severity of the defect both on 24-2 and 10-2 VF. They studied 64 eyes of 56 patients with early (54 with MD < -6 dB) or moderate (10 with MD between -6 dB and -7 dB) glaucoma, all of whom had a CVFD on the 24-2 (any of the central 12 points depressed at the < 1% or < 0.5% level on TD or PD probability plot). This study pointed out that the clinical characteristics of PFS on 10-2 VF varied significantly depending on the threshold sensitivity and magnitude of sensitivity loss or defect value at abnormal 24-2 VF test points depressed < 1%.[1]

This study concluded that threshold sensitivity and magnitude of sensitivity loss at abnormal central 12 points depressed < 1% as well as their location and number within the central-most 4 or paracentral 8 points may determine the severity of CVFDs on 24-2 VF and related PFS on 10-2 VF in glaucomatous eyes.

Wu *et al.* compared the performance of the PSD values derived from the central 12 locations of the 24–2 VF test (C24-2) to the entire 10-2 test for detecting central VF abnormalities in eyes with suspected or at risk of having glaucoma.[5] They observed that the sensitivity of the 10-2 and C24-2 PSD values was not significantly different between the 10-2 and C24-2 at matched specificities (35.9% and 35.4%, respectively; $P = 0.900$). They found a substantial agreement between the cases detected by both methods (kappa = 0.80 ± 0.04). According to their results, it can be inferred that using PSD values, the 10-2 and 24-2 tests identified a similar number of eyes having central VF abnormalities.

2. A brief note on variability of threshold sensitivity and the probability representation

The normal range of sensitivity is higher in the periphery than in the center of the field. Again, sensitivity is higher superiorly than inferiorly. A depression of 5 dB from age-normal values is considered abnormal and is also statistically significant near the center of the field. However, such deviation is totally within the normal range of sensitivity in the periphery of the test area.

Therefore, normal fluctuation across the VF is not uniformly allocated. Hence, it is not possible to use the same numerical cut-off value for all VF locations to differentiate between normal and abnormal VF test points. For this reason, in order to clinically distinguish between normal and abnormal VF locations and to identify localized defects, the probability representation is used. The probability representation uses symbols that are associated with the statistical distribution of normative data. In particular, they show the probability that a given sensitivity threshold would be obtained at the respective location for a person with a normal VF that is the same age as the patient.

3. Probability representation in TD and PD plots

The TD probability plots highlight test point locations that are significantly less sensitive than normal. It displays the difference at each test point between the patient's measured threshold sensitivity and the median normal value for the patient's age. The TD plot has 2 parts: a table of numeric values and a probability plot. The numeric value indicates the actual dB deviation from the age normal and the probability plot shows symbols that denote the statistical significance of each measured deviation.[6] Such deviations are underlined when they are worse than $P < 5\%$, 2%, 1%, and < 0.5%, of sensitivities in normal subjects who are of the same age as the patient's.[6]

The role of the PD plot is to identify localized defects. This plot shows sensitivity losses after adjusting the threshold values to remove any generalized depression or elevation of the overall hill of vision.[6] The adjustment is made based on the threshold determined at a representative point in the least diseased portion of the VF and its deviation from the age-normal threshold value for that point.[6] The PD plot uses the same symbols as the TD plot to recognize points differing by statistically significant amounts from the range of values usually found in healthy subjects. The PD plot can underline the subtle localized loss while mostly overlooking cataract effects.

4. Factors determining the occurrence of PFS on the 10-2 VF

4.1. Factors related to functional parameters

- Probability scores at abnormal 24-2 VF points within the central 10° of the TD and/or PD plot (Fig. 7-1).[4]
- Threshold sensitivity and magnitude of sensitivity loss at abnormal 24-2 VF points within the central 10° of the TD and/or PD plot (Fig. 7-1).[1]
- PSD value of 24-2 VF.[4]

4.2. Factors related to structural parameters

- The minimum mGCIPL thickness is significantly related to the presence of PFS on 10-2 VF.[4]

5. Probability symbol at the abnormal 24-2 VF points and PFS on 10-2 VF

Park *et al.* recommended that evaluating glaucomatous eyes with any abnormal central 24-2 VF points (depressed < 0.5%) by the 10-2 test would be a useful addition to the 24-2 test for an exact diagnosis and appropriate management (Figs. 7-1 and 7-2A-C).[4]

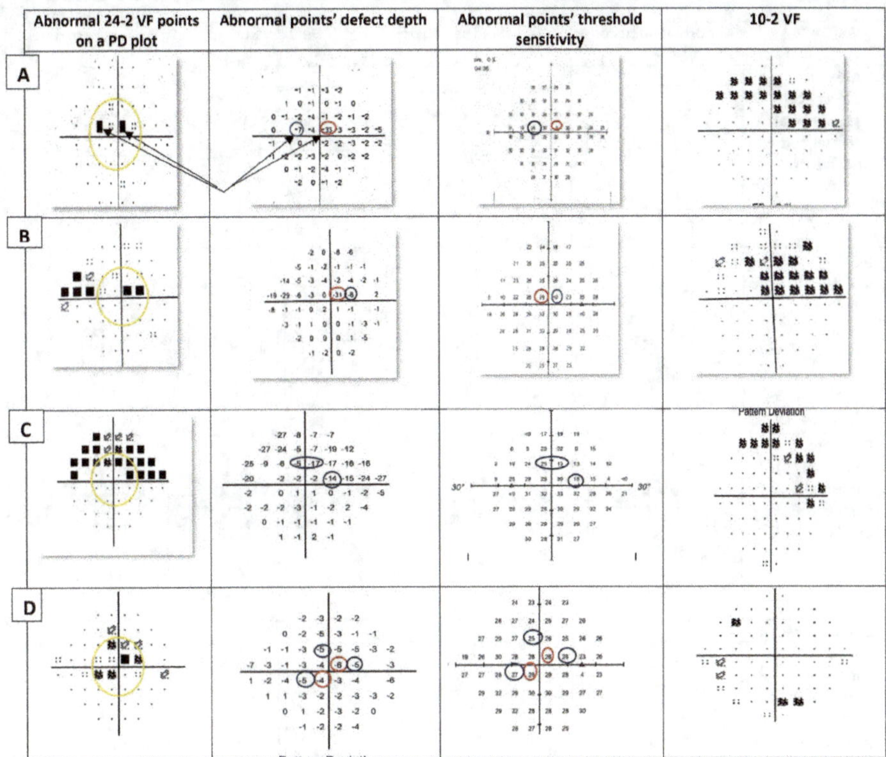

Fig. 7-1. Example of cases with abnormal 24-2 VF points within the central 12 points and related 10-2 VF defects. **(First column)** Abnormal central 24-2 VF points **(orange circle)** on a PD plot. **(Second column)** Defect depth of abnormal points. **(Third column)** Threshold sensitivity of abnormal points. The central 12 points **(orange circle)** are divided into the central-most 4 points and paracentral 8 points. Any abnormal central-most points are marked with red circle and paracentral points are markrd with blue circle in the 2nd and 3rd column. The 4th column shows PFS on 10-2 VF related to abnormal 24-2 VF points. **(A)** An IPFS with 1 abnormal point (< 0.5%) within the central-most 4 and 1 inside the paracentral 8 points on 24-2 VF. The defect is severe at the abnormal central-most point with a threshold sensitivity of 0 dB and defect value of -33 dB. The 10-2 VF test displays a superior deep arcuate scotoma. **(B)** CVFD with severe defect at an abnormal central-most point (< 0.5%) and mild defect at a paracentral point (< 0.5%). Related 10-2 VF shows a superior deep arcuate scotoma. **(C)** The 24-2 VF has no abnormalities within the central-most 4 points but has 3 abnormal paracentral points. Paracentral defects are mild to moderate, and the 10-2 VF displays a superior shallow arcuate scotoma. **(D)** The 24-2 VF has 2 central and 3 paracentral abnormal points; all are mild defects and the 10-2 VF displays only a cluster defect. This figure demonstrates that the incidence of PFS on a 10-2 test may be better predicted by measuring perimetric parameters (threshold sensitivity and defect value) at abnormal 24-2 VF points rather than only by the probability symbol of abnormal points. Reproduced from Chakravarti *et al.*[1]

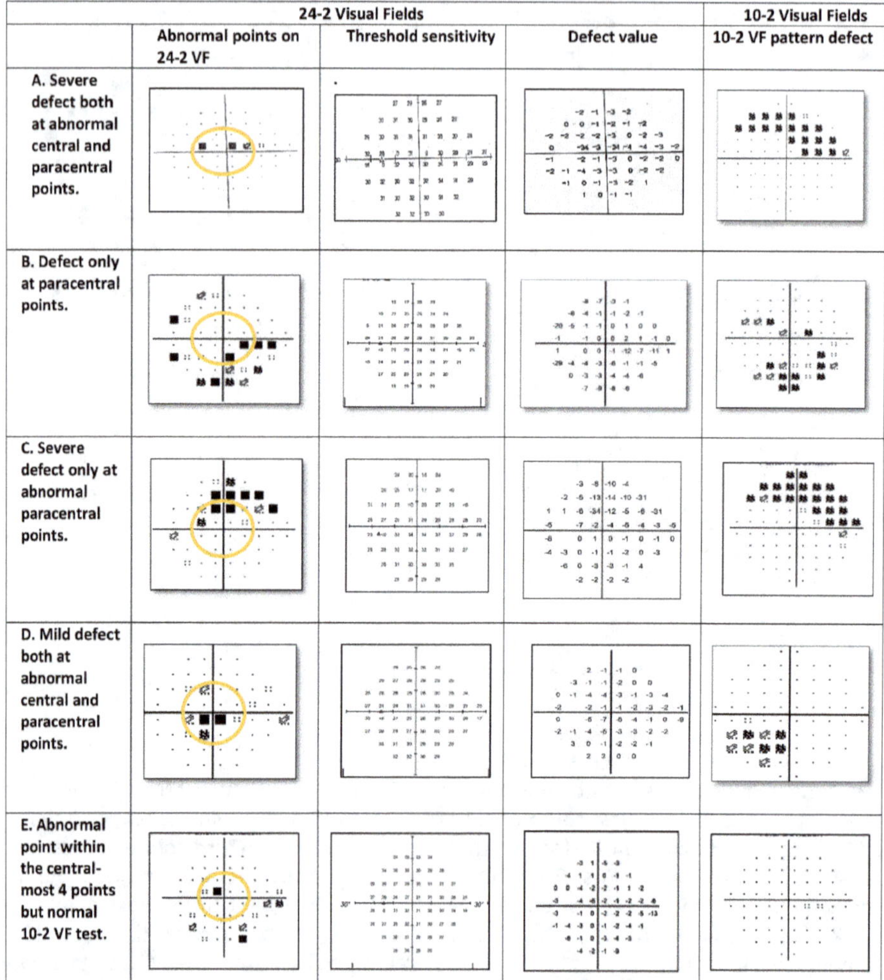

24-2 Visual Fields			10-2 Visual Fields
Abnormal points on 24-2 VF	Threshold sensitivity	Defect value	10-2 VF pattern defect
A. Severe defect both at abnormal central and paracentral points.			
B. Defect only at paracentral points.			
C. Severe defect only at abnormal paracentral points.			
D. Mild defect both at abnormal central and paracentral points.			
E. Abnormal point within the central-most 4 points but normal 10-2 VF test.			

Fig. 7-2. Representative cases of abnormal 24-2 VF points within the central 12 points and related PFS on 10-2 VF. The presence of abnormal central 24-2 VF points demonstrates the predictive value of having arcuate-like scotoma on 10-2 VFs. **(First column)** Mentions the location location of abnormal points (central or paracentral) on the 24-2 VF. **(Second column)** A PD plot with abnormal points on the 24-2 VF **(orange circle)**. **(Third column)** The threshold value at an abnormal point. **(Fourth column)** The amount of sensitivity loss or defect value at an abnormal point. **(Fifth column)** Scotoma on 10-2 VF. **(A-E)** Abnormal 24-2 VF points depressed < 0.5% either within the central-most 4 points or paracentral 8 points or having both within the central 10°. However, only **(A-C)** display arcuate-like PFS on 10-2 VF. In **(D)**, the 10-2 VF demonstrates only a cluster defect. Further, in **(E)** the 10-2 VF does not show any defect at all despite the presence of an abnormal 24-2 point depressed < 0 .5% within the central 5°. Reproduced from Chakravarti *et al.*[1]

However, they also reported that 10% of eyes with abnormal 24-2 VF points depressed to < 0.5% within the central-most 4 points, and 30% of eyes within the paracentral 8 points did not display any PFS on the 10-2 VF test.[4] Similarly, Chakravarti *et al.* observed that 15.6% of eyes with abnormal 24-2 VF points depressed to < 1% either within the central-most 4 points or paracentral 8 points did not demonstrate any PFS or cluster defect on the 10-2 VF test (Fig. 7-2D, 7-2E).[1] Altogether, these findings suggest that the presence of any abnormal 24-2 VF point depressed < 1% (probability representation) within the central 12 points cannot always ensure the occurrence of PFS on 10-2 VF test (Fig. 7-2E). Therefore, the probability score at abnormal central VF points on 24-2 VF does not provide adequate information on the occurrence of PFS on the 10-2 VF test. The probability score may not fully explain the occurrence of PFS on the 10-2 test (Figs. 7-1, 7-2).[1]

6. Threshold sensitivity at abnormal 24-2 VF points and PFS on 10-2 VF

Several investigators have reported a strong association between the depressed threshold sensitivity (Figure 7-2 third column) at abnormal central 24-2 VF points and corresponding PFS on the 10-2 VF (Fig. 7-2 fifth column).[1] It has been also indicated that an association between the magnitude of sensitivity loss (defect value) at abnormal 24-2 VF points within the central 10° (Fig. 7-2 fifth column) and corresponding PFS on the 10-2 VF (Fig. 7-2 fourth column).[1] The incidence of PFS on a 10-2 test may be better predicted by measuring perimetric parameters at abnormal 24-2 VF points rather than by only the probability symbol of abnormal points (Figs. 7-1, 7-2).[1]

7. PSD value on 24-2 VF test and PFS on 10-2 VF

In recent times, more investigators have examined the relationship between the PSD value of the 24-2 VF test and PFS on 10-2 VF.[4,5] It has been observed that among the existing standard metrics of VF, PSD is a better indicator than MD for the presence of PFS on the 10-2 VF test in early glaucoma.[4,5] On the 24-2 VF test, eyes with similar MD but with a greater PSD show PFS on the 10-2 VF test and the PSD of the 24-2 VF test is more predictable in finding abnormalities on the 10-2 VF test compared to the MD of the 24-2 VF test

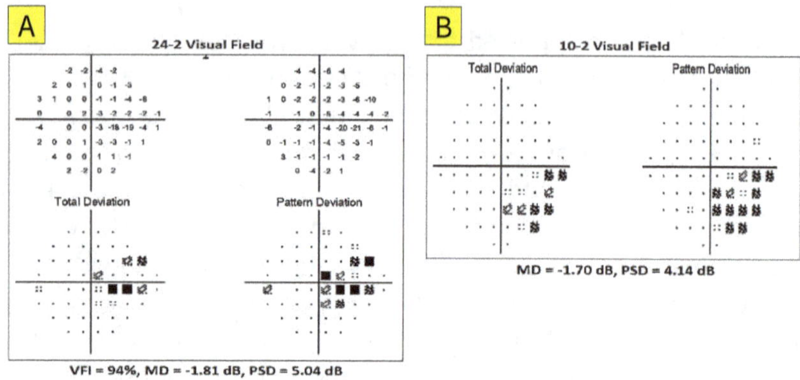

Fig. 7-3. A representative case of CVFD on 24-2 VF with a higher PSD value and related PFS on 10-2. **(A)** The left eye of a patient in the early glaucoma stage shows abnormal points depressed < 0.5% within the central 10° in the superior and inferior hemifield on the PD probability plot of the Humphrey 24-2 VF. The PSD of this 24-2 VF is 5.04 dB, which is higher than the MD value of -1.81 dB. **(B)** On the 10-2 VF test, his left eye displays an inferior arcuate-like scotoma. The frequency of PFS on the 10-2 VF test is higher in the presence of a greater PSD value than the MD value of a 24-2 VF with central abnormal points.

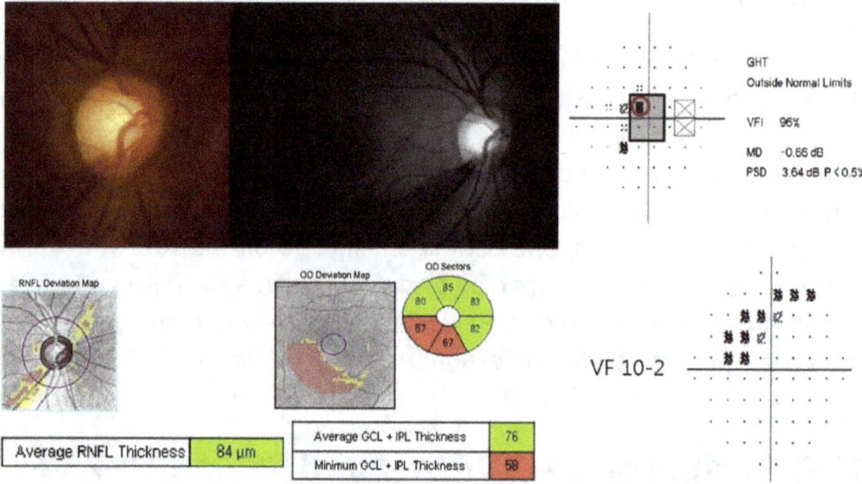

Fig. 7-4. A representative case with an abnormal VF point depressed < 0.5% within the innermost 4 points on the 24-2 VF test **(red circle)**. This case shows a PSD of 3.64 dB, which is greater than the MD of -0.66 dB on the 24-2 VF test. The abnormal 24-2 VF point within the innermost 4 points turned out to be an arcuate-like PFS on the 10-2 VF test. Reproduced from Park *et al.*[4]

(Figs. 7-3, 7-4). This finding indicates that, in early glaucoma, the prevalence of PFS on 10-2 VF is higher if the PSD value of a 24-2 VF is greater than usual even with few abnormal central points on the 24-2 VF.[4]

8. Minimum mGCIPL thickness and PFS on 10-2 VF

For identifying early glaucoma, mGCIPL thickness is reported to be the most useful among several parameters provided by the macular ganglion cell analysis (GCA) of the Cirrus OCT.[7] The combined thickness of the GCL and the IPL is termed GCIPL. It has been reported that the minimum mGCIPL thickness is more accurate than the average mGCIPL thickness for detecting early glaucoma[7] and the minimum mGCIPL thickness is strongly related to the occurrence of PFS on the 10-2 VF test among structural parameters.[4]

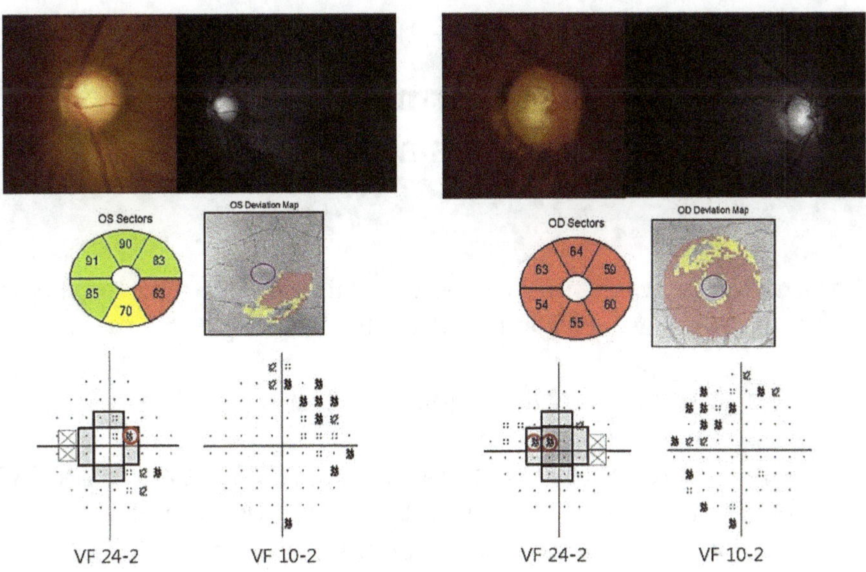

Fig. 7-5. Representative cases with abnormal VF points within the central 12 points on the Humphrey 24-2 VF test. **(Left)** The first case has only 1 < 2% depressed abnormal 24-2 VF point within the paracentral 8 points **(red circle)**. **(Right)** The latter case has 1 <2% depressed point within the innermost 4 points and another < 2% depressed point within the paracentral 8 points **(red circles)** on the 24-2 VF test. The abnormal 24-2 VF points spatially correlate with the thinning of the GCL–IPL thickness, and these eyes had PFS on the 10-2 VF test. Reproduced from Park *et al.*[4]

Investigators observe that the GCA algorithm of the Cirrus OCT can successfully measure the thickness of the mGCIPL with excellent reproducibility.[8,9]

Recent research has observed that in glaucomatous eyes minimum mGCIPL thickness and any central 12 points depressed < 0.5% on 24-2 VF, and any central 12 points depressed < 5% on 24-2 VF that spatially correspond to mGCIPL thinning are related factors to the presence of PFS on 10-2 VF.[4] They underscored that in glaucomatous eyes with any abnormal central 24-2 VF points depressed < 5% (even if a point is not depressed < 0.5%), having a spatial correlation to the mGCIPL thinning map, that correlation points to the presence of PFS on the 10-2 VF test. The incidence of minimum mGCIPL thicknesses depressed < 1% is higher in eyes with PFS in comparison to eyes without PFS.[4]

Figure 7-5 presents representative cases with abnormal 24-2 VF points spatially correlated with the thinning of mGCIPL thickness and PFS on the 10-2 VF test.[4]

9. Clinical clues for determining the characteristics of PFS on a 10-2 VF using a 24-2 VF

The factors linked with abnormal 24-2 VF points that determine the characteristics and severity of PFS on 10-2 VF are the following:

- The threshold sensitivity (dB) value at any central 12 points depressed < 1% on 24-2 VF.
- The deviated threshold sensitivity value (dB) at any central 12 points depressed < 1% on 24-2 VF on TD and PD plots.
- The location of any central 12 points depressed < 1% on 24-2 VF in a hemifield.
- The percentage and number of central 12 points depressed < 1% on 24-2 VF in a hemifield.

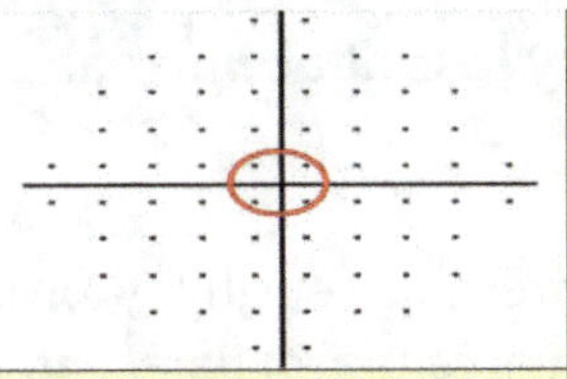

24-2 test pattern. Central-most 4 points are outlined with red circle within central 5°.

Evaluating the severity of functional damage in glaucomatous eyes, HPA classification takes into account the presence of abnormalities within the central 5° of the 24-2 grid.

- In early disease stage, a glaucomatous visual field must have a sensitivity of at least 15dB at all test points in the central 5°;

- In moderate disease stage may have a sensitivity of <15dB in a test point within 5° of fixation, only in one hemifield;

- In severe disease stage may have a test point within the central 5° with a sensitivity of < 15dB in both hemifields;

- Any glaucomatous VF can be classified as a severe defect if any one test point in the central 5° has a sensitivity of 0dB.

Fig. 7-6. The HPA system classifies eyes with MD ≤ -6 dB as severe if the damage is located within the central 5° of the 24-2 VF and identifies the threshold sensitivity cut-off value at 15 dB at abnormal test points in the central 5°.

10. Defects are considered severe when the threshold sensitivity value is below 15 dB

Some investigators have pointed out that clinically, threshold values below 15–19 dB should be interpreted with caution, as they may not be reliable for assessing the true level of damage or glaucomatous progression.[10] To evaluate the severity of functional damage in glaucomatous eyes, Hodapp, Parrish, and Anderson's (HPA) classification takes into account the presence of abnormalities within the central 5° of the 24-2 grid and determines 15 dB as the cut-off value of threshold sensitivity at abnormal test points in the central 5° (see Chapter 4).[11,12] The HPA system classifies eyes with MD ≤-6 dB as severe if the damage is located within the central 5° and the threshold sensitivity at a test point < 15 dB within the central 5° in both hemifields of the 24-2 VF. The HPA classification system (see Chapter 5) recommends the following criteria as mentioned and described in Figure 7-6.

11. Threshold sensitivity (dB) and sensitivity loss at abnormal 24-2 VF points and PFS on 10-2 VF

A significant association was observed between threshold sensitivity lower than 20 dB and sensitivity loss < -15 dB at an abnormal central or paracentral test point on the 24-2 VF and arcuate-like scotoma on the 10-2 VF.[1] In a study on the prediction of PFS on 10-2 VF by central 24-2 defects, Chakravarti *et al.* observed that an arcuate scotoma on the 10-2 VF test was more likely when a central-most point on the 24-2 had a threshold sensitivity below 20 dB (OR, 7.2; 95% CI, 1.7–30.1, P = 0.002).[1]

Again, in early glaucomatous eyes, the higher risk of having arcuate-like scotoma on 10-2 VF is increased when the magnitude of sensitivity loss (defect value) is worse than −15 dB at any abnormal central or paracentral test point on 24-2 VF (OR, 8.0; 95% CI, 1.5–41.6, P = 0.005).[1]

Moreover, the risk of having deep arcuate scotoma on 10-2 VF is significantly increased in the presence of a high magnitude of sensitivity loss (> -34 dB) at any abnormal central 12 points on 24-2 VF.[1] However, the incidence of such PFS on 10-2 VF is much lower in the presence of such abnormalities within the paracentral 8 points.[1]

12. The relative position of abnormal 24-2 VF points and PFS on 10-2 VF

The location of abnormal 24 VF points in each hemifield can also predict the severity of PFS on 10-2 VF.[1] Several investigators have reported that an abnormal superior nasal point defect (< 1%) in the central 5° on 24-2 VF is significantly associated with an arcuate defect on 10-2 VF (OR, 4.6; 95% CI, 1.5–13.7; P = 0.004).[1] However, the incidence of arcuate scotoma on 10-2 VF is much lower when a paracentral point is affected or any abnormal central 24-2 VF point is located superior temporally in the central 5°.[1]

13. Comparing the severity of superior and inferior PFS on the 10-2 VF

The severity of superior and inferior PFS on the 10-2 VF test is not the same regarding the depth and threat to fixation. Figure 7-7 depicts a case that exemplifies the severity of a superior PFS on the 10-2 VF with greater defect depth (worse MD and PSD) and more abnormal 10-2 points within 5° of fixation when compared to another case having the inferior PFS on 10-2 VF, as shown in Figure 7-8. However, the 24-2 VF shown in Figure 7-7D fulfils all the conditions of risk factors that contribute to having a deep arcuate PFS on 10-2 VF (Fig. 7-7E, 7-7F) related to abnormal 24-2 VF points within the central 5° and 10° (as mentioned in Section 14 of the present chapter). The main difference between these 2 PFS on the 10-2 VF is that the superior PFS (Fig. 7-7E, 7-7F) corresponds to a defect within the central-most 4 points on the 24-2 VF (Fig. 7-7D) while the inferior PFS (Fig. 7-8E) corresponds to a defect within the paracentral 8 points on the 24-2 VF (Fig. 7-8B).[13]

- Classic arcuate scotomas, including those that extend into the central 10°, are more often seen in the superior hemifield.[3]
- The average TD values and the number of abnormal points revealed superior VF defects on 10-2 VF are deeper and closer to fixation than those in the inferior VF (Figs. 7-7E, 7-7F, 7-8E).[3]
- Superior defects specifically have greater defect depth (worse MD and PSD) and more abnormal 10-2 points within 5° of fixation (Fig. 7-7E, 7-7F) when compared to inferior 10-2 defects (Fig. 7-8E).[3]
- Superior 10-2 VF loss may have greater potential for functional disability than inferior 10-2 VF loss.[3]

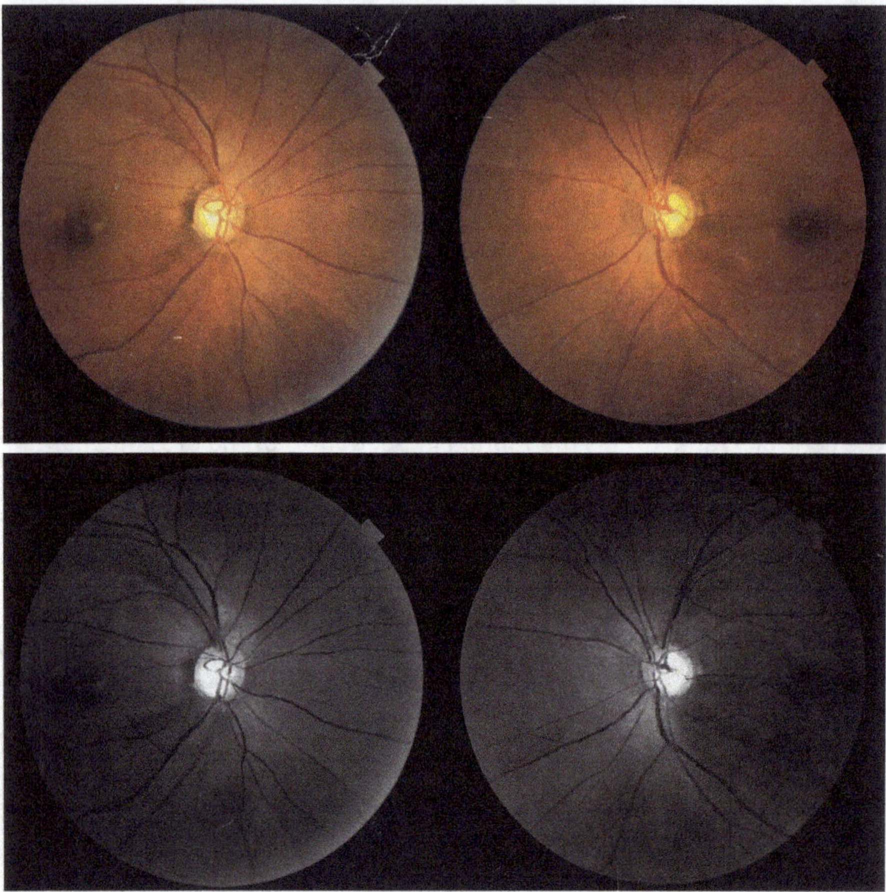

Fig. 7-7. The severity of superior PFS on 10-2 VF. This patient was diagnosed with bilateral NTG in 2013. He had been using latanoprost and a fixed combination of brinzolamide and brimonidine tartrate ophthalmic suspension in both eyes since his diagnosis. On the VF test he presented with advanced loss in the right eye. The MD slope in the left eye was not significant until 2018 (-0.22 ± 0.48 dB/year). However, a recent follow-up detected progressive VF changes in the left eye and the patient was referred for further evaluation. Best-corrected visual acuity was 20/20 (0.0 logMAR) bilaterally and IOP was 11 mmHg and 13 mmHg in the right and left eye, respectively. **(A)** Fundus photograph in 2014 showing an absence of inferior neuroretinal rim over more than 45° in his right eye and disc would be graded as stage 7 as per disc damage likelihood scale (DDLS). In the left eye, superior and inferior neuroretinal rim thinning is noticed and rim/disc ratio is less than 0.1 inferiorly as per DDLS grading. **(B)** The red-free fundus photographs of both eyes demonstrate superotemporal and inferotemporal RNFL defects.

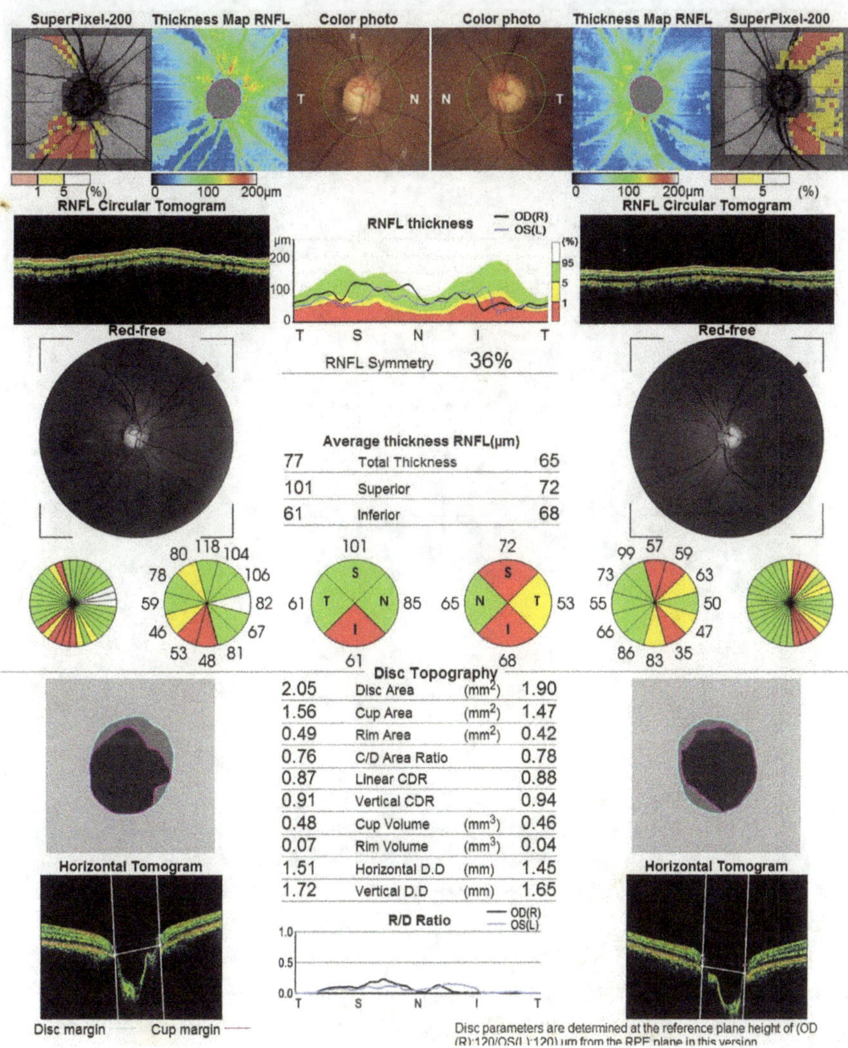

Fig. 7-7. Continued. **(C)** The OCT performed in 2013 showed the following parameters for the right and left eye, respectively: average RNFL thickness of 77 µm and 65 µm, average superior RNFL thickness of 101 µm and 72 µm, and inferior RNFL thickness of 61 µm and 68 µm.

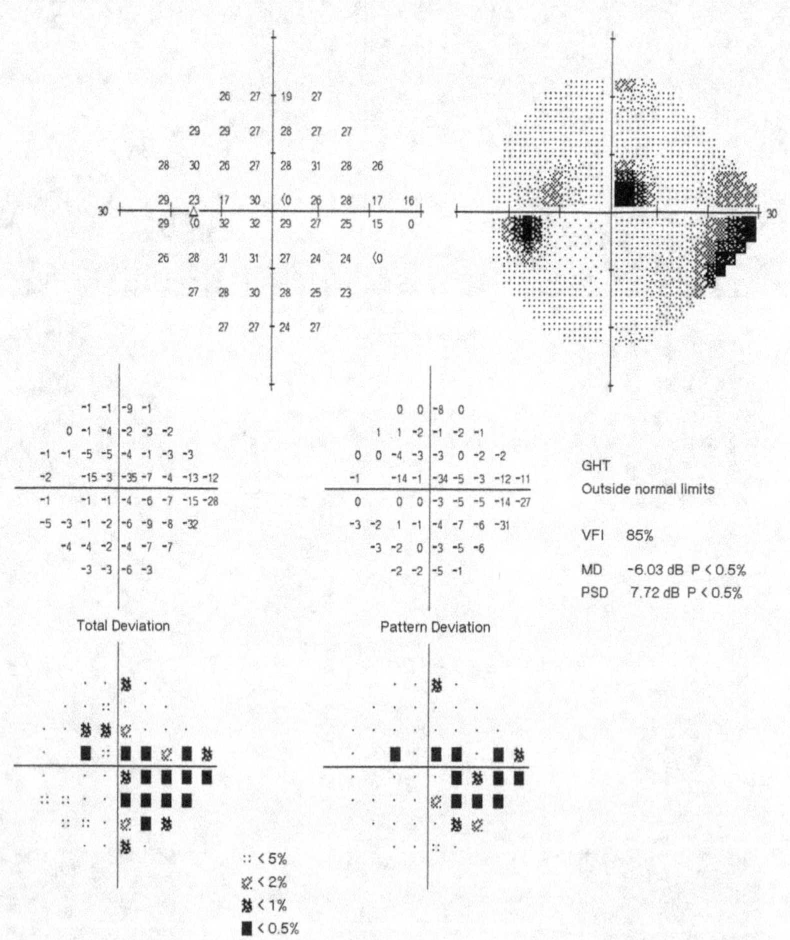

Fig. 7-7. Continued. **(D)** The patient's left-eye VF demonstrates a central defect in the superior hemifield and nasal field defects both in the superior and inferior hemifields (VFI 85%, MD -6.03 dB, and PSD 7.72 dB). The central defect in the left eye presents an abnormal point *P* < 0.5%, within the central 5° with very low threshold sensitivity (< 0 dB) and depressed uniformly on the TD and PD probability plots with a defect value of -34 dB in the superior nasal hemifield. Two abnormal paracentral points in the superior hemifield, and 1 in the inferior hemifield within the central 10° are noticed. Calculating the risk factor of having PFS on the 10-2 VF related to defects on abnormal 24-2VF points can be predicted per location, threshold sensitivity, and defect value of these abnormal points. However, the severity and magnitude of the CVFD is poorly represented by the 24-2 VF. In a busy clinical practice, the implication of such a defect can often be underestimated by a 24-2 VF test alone.

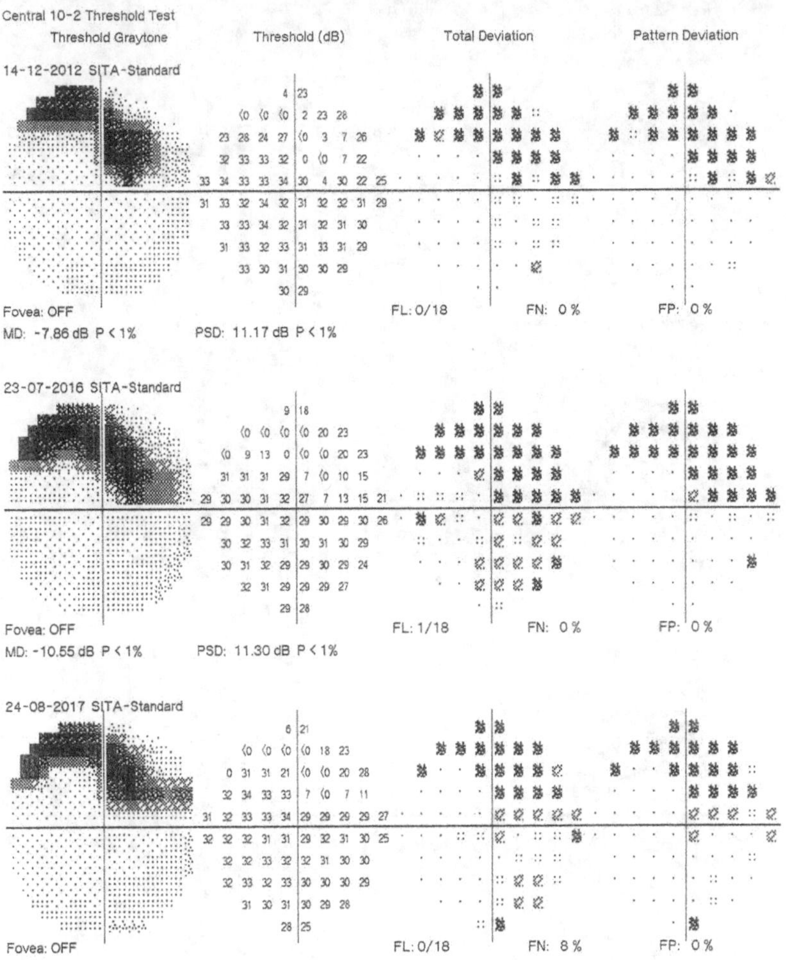

Fig. 7-7. Continued. **(E)** In contrast to the 24-2 VF, the 10-2 VF demonstrates a deep arcuate scotoma in the superior hemifield and illustrates the extent of central VF loss. Since 2012, the overview printout of the 10-2 VF always indicated the severity of the patient's central VF loss in 2 ways: first, by showing higher MD and PSD values of PFS on 10-2 than the 24-2 VF and second, by showing the abnormal 10-2 points within 5° of fixation. Please note that this case shows a superior PFS on the 10-2VF test that was not evident on the 24-2VF test (comparable to Fig. 2-7).

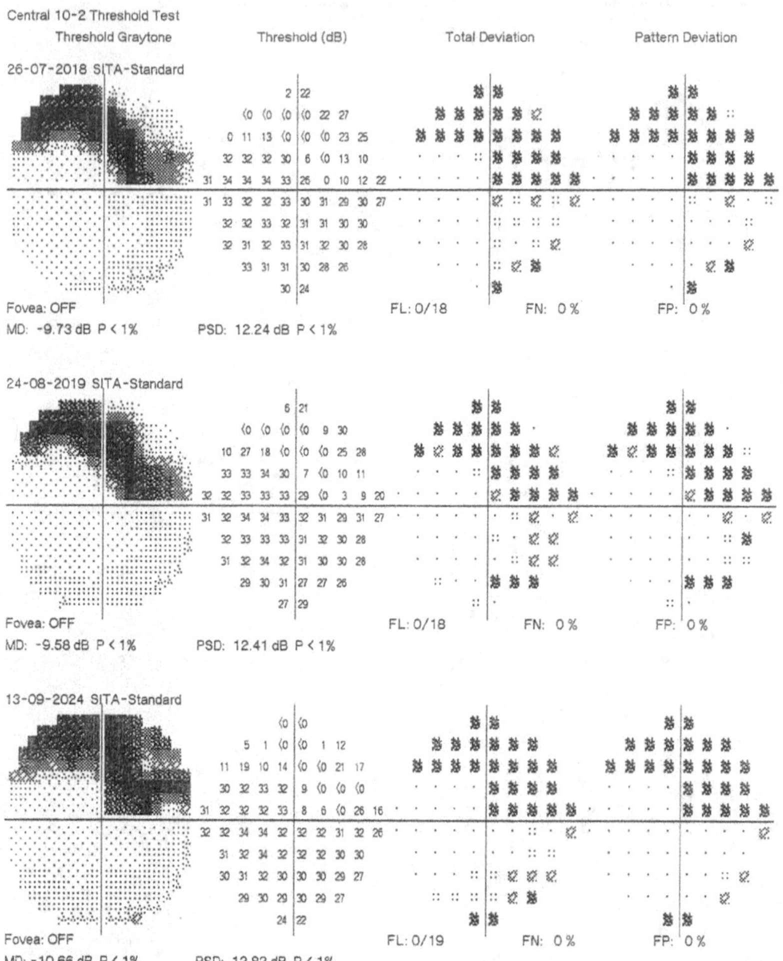

Fig. 7-7. Continued. **(F)** This overview printout of a 10-2 VF indicates the severity of the patient's central VF loss from 2018 to 2024 in his left eye. In 2024, the values were MD -10.66 dB and PSD 12.82dB on the 10-2 VF.

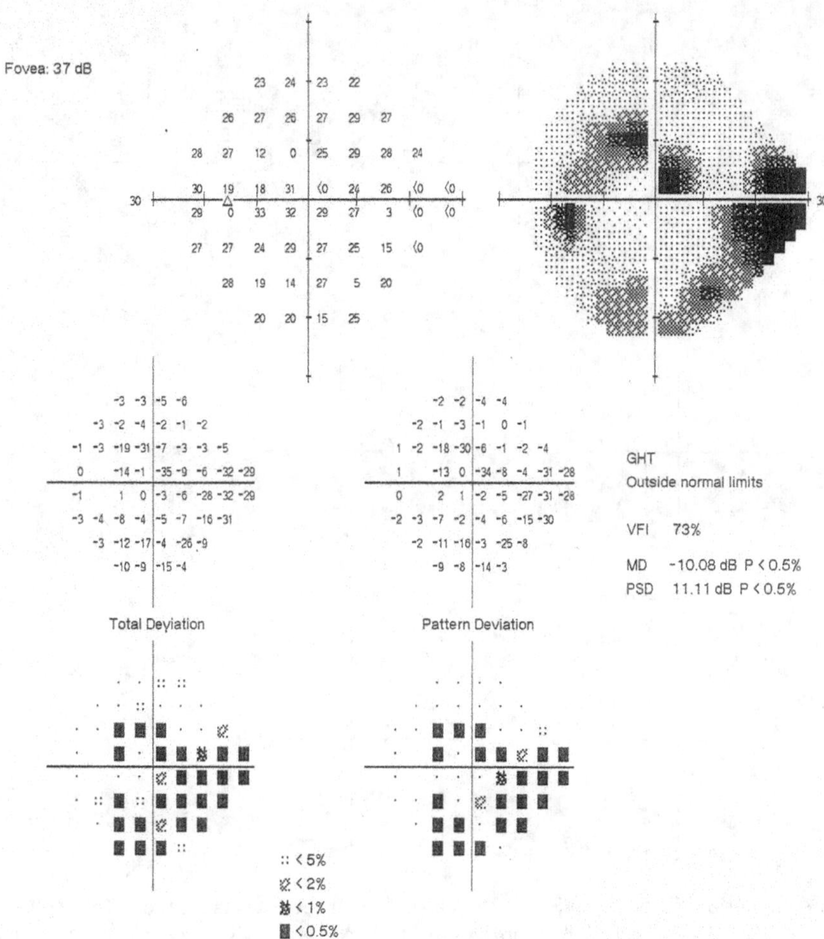

Fig. 7-7. Continued. **(G)** The patient's most recent 24-2 VF of the left eye records the deterioration of the VF with a central defect with MD -10.08 dB and PSD 11.11 dB.

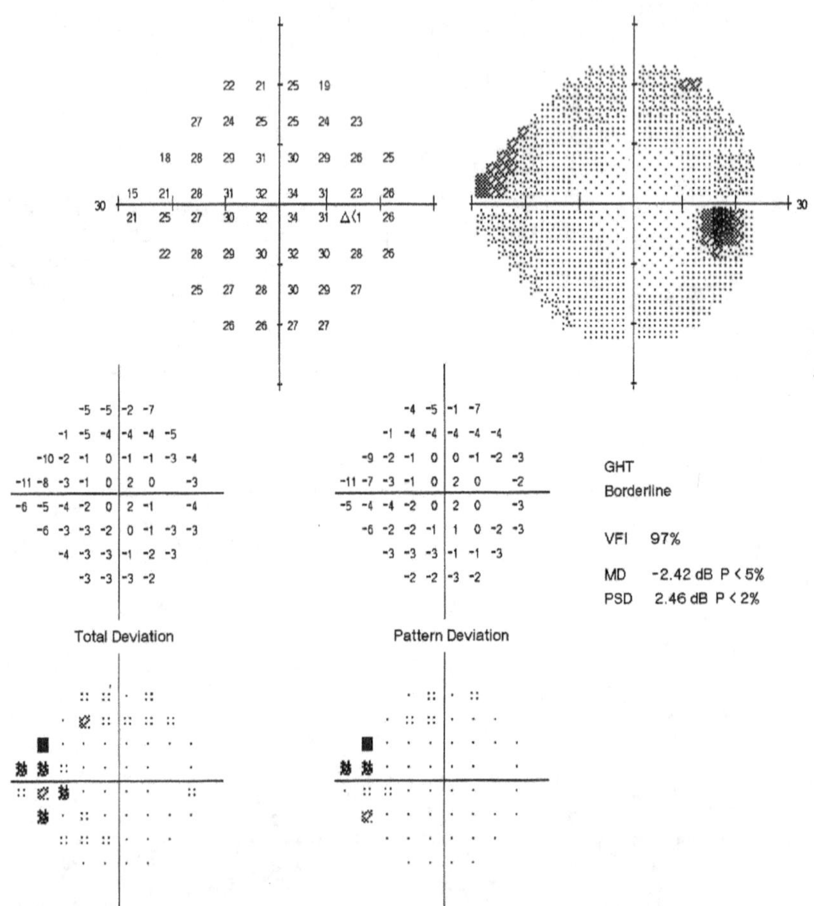

Fig. 7-8. Inferior PFS on 10-2 VF. This 70-year-old male patient was diagnosed with bilateral POAG in 2020. On a recent follow-up visit, his best-corrected visual acuity was 20/30 (0.20 logMAR) and 20/20 (0.0 logMAR) in the right and left eye, respectively. He had been using latanoprost eye drops in both eyes since his diagnosis. IOP was well controlled with medical treatment at 12 mmHg and 13 mmHg in the right and left eye, respectively. His 24-2 VF in early 2021 **(A)** showed a superior nasal step in the right eye and **(B)** an early arcuate scotoma in the inferior hemifield of the left eye. According to the severity classification, his left eye VF demonstrated an early moderate field defect with MD -6.37 dB, PSD 7.44 dB, and VFI 88%. The left eye VF showed only 1 abnormal point depressed < 0.5% within the 8 paracentral points. The threshold sensitivity and defect depth of that abnormal paracentral point was 15 dB.

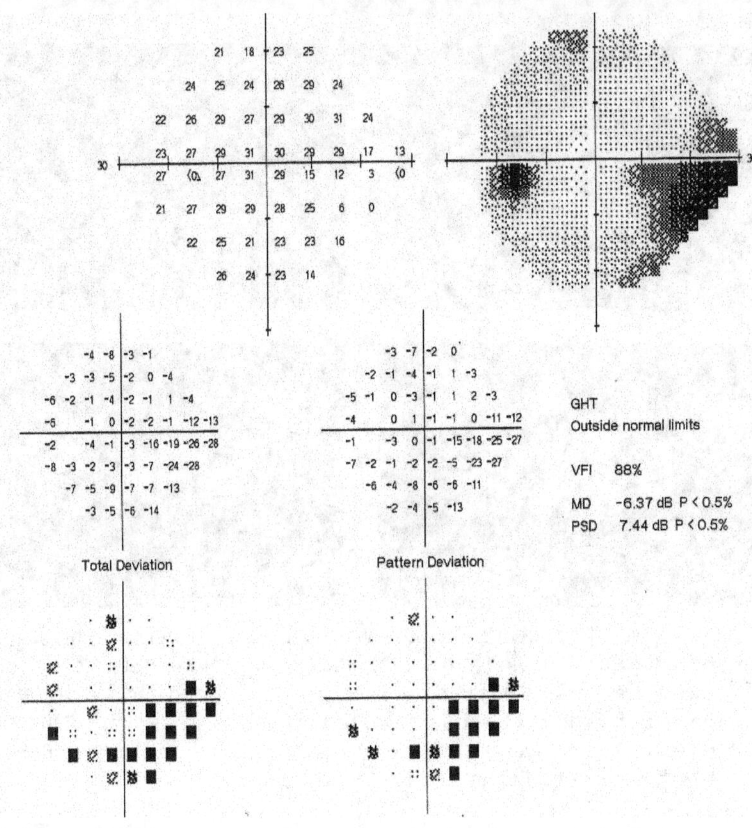

Fig. 7-8. Continued. **(B)**

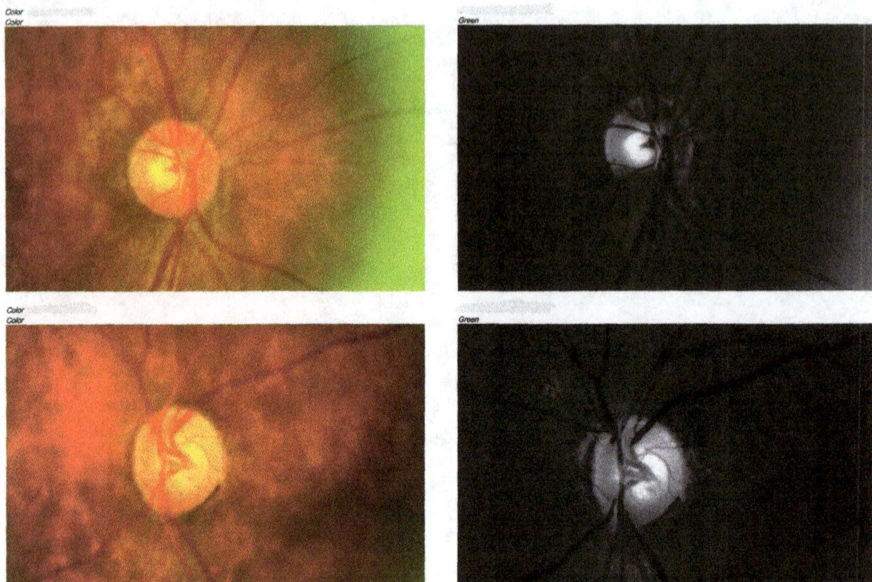

Fig. 7-8. Continued. The patient's VF results were in good agreement with his **(C)** optic disc photograph and **(D)** OCT findings from 2021, showing a borderline superotemporal RNFL defect in the right eye as well as temporal and superotemporal defects in the left eye. The RNFL parameters for the right and left eye, respectively, were: average RNFL thickness of 103.4 μm and 85.1 μm, average superior RNFL thickness of 90.4 μm and 68.8 μm, and inferior RNFL thickness of 116.3 μm and 101.3 μm.

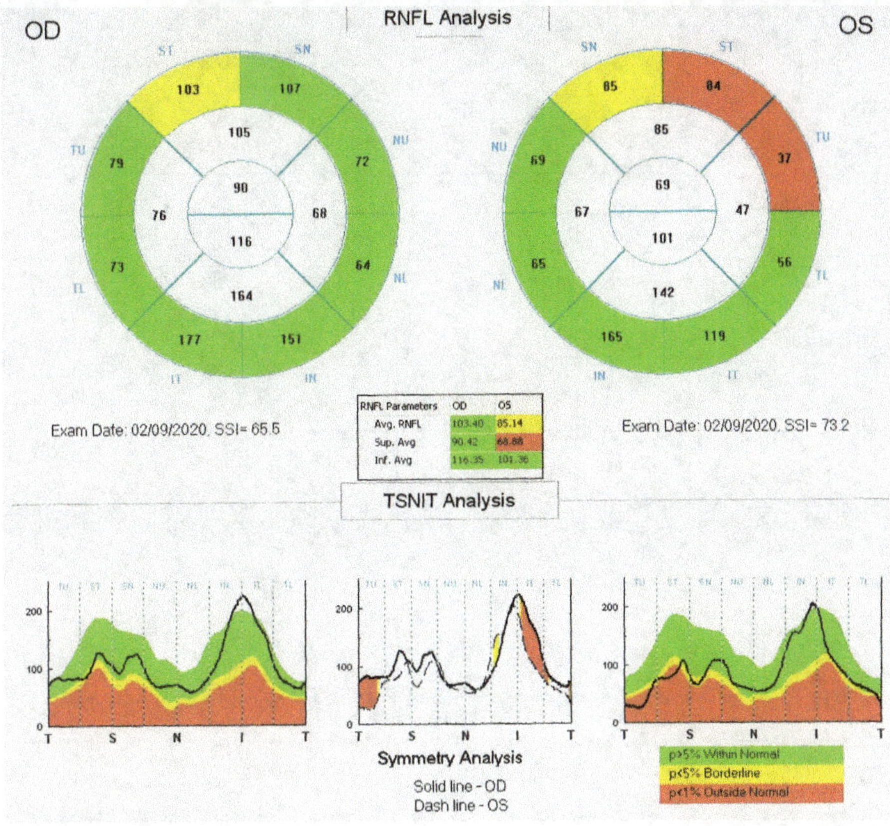

RNFL Parameters	OD	OS
Avg. RNFL	103.40	85.14
Sup. Avg	90.42	68.88
Inf. Avg	116.35	101.36

Fig. 7-8. Continued. **(D)**

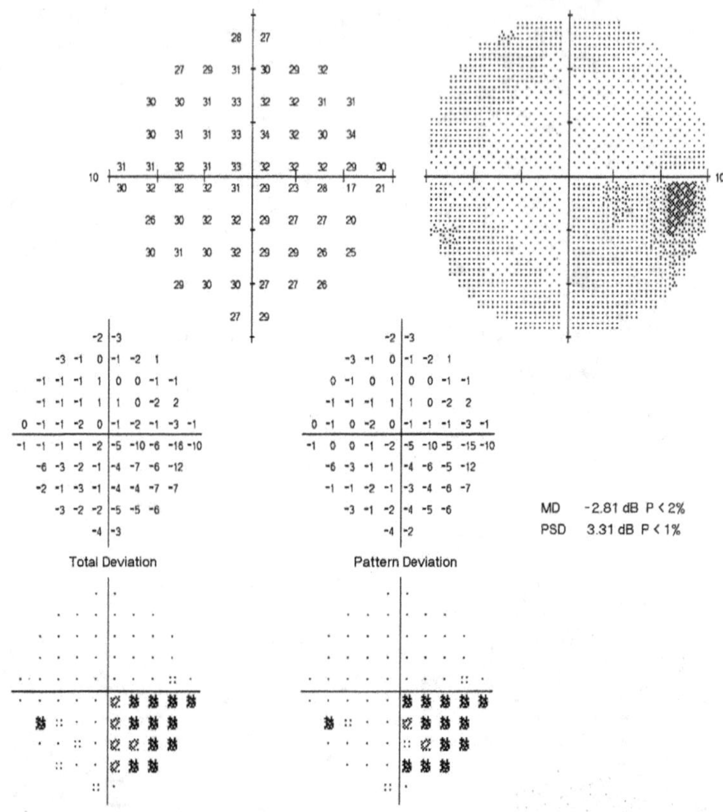

Total Deviation

Pattern Deviation

MD   −2.81 dB P < 2%
PSD 3.31 dB P < 1%

Fig. 7-8. Continued. **(E)** After 10-2 VF testing, the patient's left eye demonstrated an inferior PFS, representing the true extent of VF loss that reflects the actual severity of the CVFD in the left eye. The CVFD on 10-2 VF was closer to fixation, which was not reflected by the 24-2 VF.

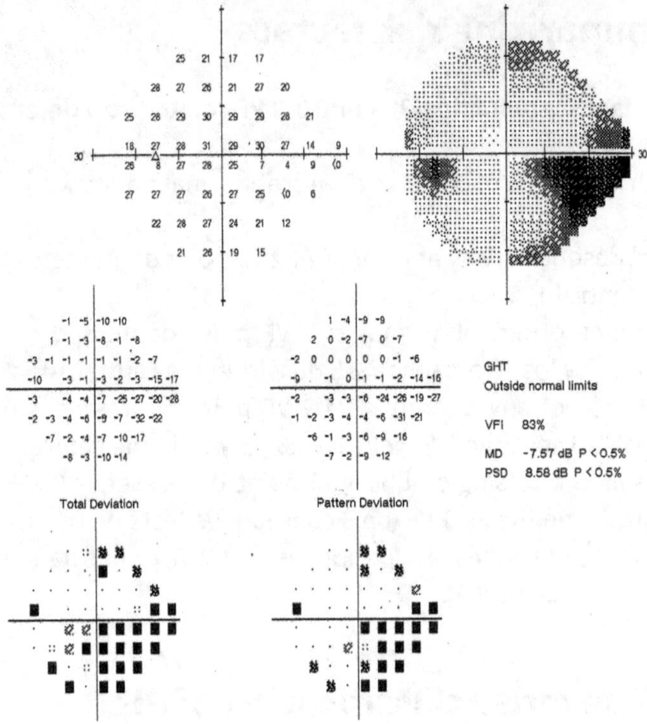

Fig. 7-8. Continued. **(F)** However, the most recent 24-2 VF, performed in August 2024, detected an abnormal point within the central-most 4 points. The 10-2 VF test detected this central defect in the patient's left eye 3 years ahead of the 24-2 VF test.

14. Summarizing risk factors

14.1. Risk factors of having PFS on 10-2 VF related to a defect in central 10° on 24-2 VF

- High PSD value of the 24-2 VF with abnormal points within the central 10°.
- The presence of any abnormal 24-2 VF point depressed < 0.5% within the central 10°.
- Presence of any abnormal 24-2 VF point depressed < 0.5% with a sensitivity loss worse than -15 dB within the central 10°.
- Presence of any abnormal 24-2 VF point depressed < 0.5% with a threshold sensitivity lower than 20 dB within the central 10°.
- Presence of a single abnormal point depressed < 0.5% within the central 5°on the 24-2 VF (on 3 consecutive tests on the same point).
- Presence of abnormal superior nasal 24-2 VF points depressed < 0.5% within the central 5°.

15. The severity classification of PFS

Because of the clinical importance of central vision, more information is needed regarding the possible impact of PFS on a patient's QoL. The obvious impact of an arcuate PFS on a patient's central vision is more serious than that of a cluster defect. QoL is severely affected in the presence of such deep defects. Hence, a classification system for grading the clinical characteristics of PFS on a 10-2 VF test is of utmost importance for understanding the influence of different types of PFS on a patient's visual function and functional vision. The severity of PFS on 10-2 VFs is divided into 3 groups based on the characteristics of pattern defects (Table 7-1).[1]

For evaluating the severity of PFS on 10-2 VF, some studies recorded the number of abnormal 10-2 points within 5° of fixation to examine the fixation threat based on hemispheric defect location (Fig. 7-9).[3] They also applied MD and PSD values of the 10-2 VF for severity classifications, as shown in Figure 7-9.

Table 7-1. The severity classification of PFS on 10-2 VF based on pattern of defects[1]

Severity of defect	Characteristics
Severe defect	Deep and shallow arcuate defects and horizontal step defects are considered severe forms of pattern defects with profound functional loss. Functional loss is greater (worse MD and PSD value) in an arcuate group than in the non-arcuate group on 10-2 VF.
Moderate defect	The severity of the partial arcuate type of pattern defect is considered a moderate loss.
Minimal defect	Cluster defects are interpreted as a minimum defect.

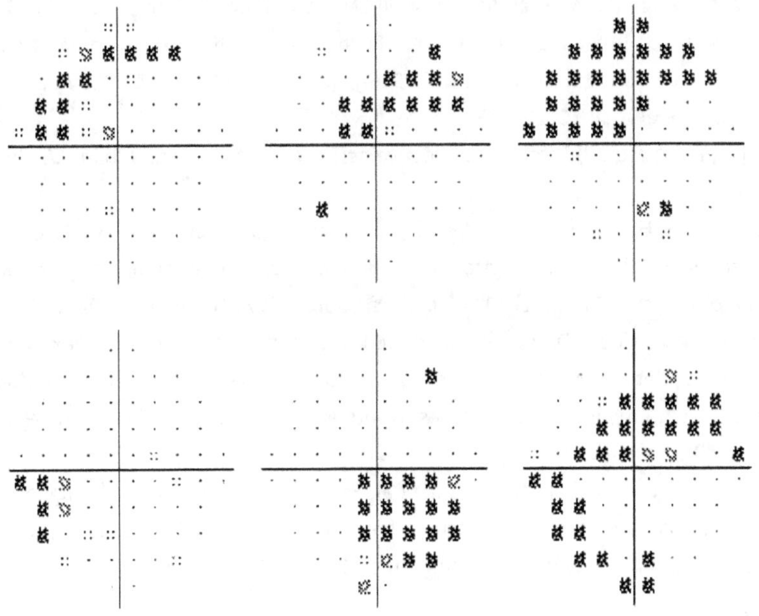

Fig. 7-9. The severity of PFS on 10-2 VF based on the number of abnormal 10-2 points within 5° of fixation and MD and PSD values of the 10-2 VF. **(Top left)** Mild arcuate defect (MD: -3.48 dB, PSD: 2.47 dB). **(Top middle)** Moderate arcuate defect (MD: -3.80 dB, PSD: 6.33 dB). **(Top right)** Advanced arcuate defect (MD: -12.76 dB, PSD: 14.50 dB). **(Bottom left)** Nasal defect (MD: -0.85 dB, PSD: 1.75 dB). **(Bottom middle)** Temporal defect (MD: -5.02 dB, PSD: 12.19 dB). **(Bottom right)** Combined superior and inferior defect (MD: -10.90 dB, PSD: 14.18 dB). In the last plot, the superior defect involves fixation while the lower field defect spares fixation. Reproduced from Sullivan-Mee *et al.*[3]

References

1. Chakravarti T, Moghimi S, Weinreb RN. Prediction of central visual field severity in glaucoma. J Glaucoma. 2022;31(6):430-7. https://doi.org/10.1097/IJG.0000000000002031

2. West ME, Sharpe GP, Hutchison DM, et al. Value of 10-2 visual field testing in glaucoma patients with early 24-2 visual field loss. Ophthalmology. 2021;128(4):545-53. https://doi.org/10.1016/j.ophtha.2020.08.033

3. Sullivan-Mee M, Tran MT, Pensyl D, et al. Prevalence, features, and severity of glaucomatous visual field loss measured with the 10-2 achromatic threshold visual field test. Am J Ophthalmol. 2016;168:40-51. https://doi.org/10.1016/j.ajo.2016.05.003

4. Park HY, Hwang BE, Shin HY, Park CK. Clinical clues to predict the presence of parafoveal scotoma on Humphrey 10-2 visual field using a Humphrey 24-2 visual field. Am J Ophthalmol. 2016;161:150-9. https://doi.org/10.1016/j.ajo.2015.10.007

5. Wu Z, Medeiros FA, Weinreb RN, Zangwill LM. Performance of the 10-2 and 24-2 Visual Field Tests for Detecting Central Visual Field Abnormalities in Glaucoma. Am J Ophthalmol. 2018 Dec;196:10-17. doi: 10.1016/j.ajo.2018.08.010. Epub 2018 Aug 10. PMID: 30099037; PMCID: PMC6258276.

6. Heijl A, Bengtsson B, Patella VM. Effective perimetry. 4th Edition. Dublin, CA: Carl Zeiss Meditec; 2012.

7. Takayama K, Hangai M, Durbin M, et al. A novel method to detect local ganglion cell loss in early glaucoma using spectral-domain optical coherence tomography. Invest Ophthalmol Vis Sci. 2012;53(11):6904-13. https://doi.org/10.1167/iovs.12-10210

8. Mwanza JC, Oakley JD, Budenz DL, et al. Macular ganglion cell-inner plexiform layer: automated detection and thickness reproducibility with spectral domain-optical coherence tomography in glaucoma. Invest Ophthalmol Vis Sci. 2011;52(11):8323-9. https://doi.org/10.1167/iovs.11-7962

9. Francoz M, Fenolland JR, Giraud JM, et al. Reproducibility of macular ganglion cell-inner plexiform layer thickness measurement with cirrus HD-OCT in normal, hypertensive, and glaucomatous eyes. Br J Ophthalmol. 2014;98(3):322-8. https://doi.org/10.1136/bjophthalmol-2012-302242

10. Gardiner SK, Swanson WH, Goren D, et al. Assessment of the reliability of standard automated perimetry in regions of glaucomatous damage. Ophthalmology. 2014;121(7):1359-69. https://doi.org/10.1016/j.ophtha.2014.01.020

11. Brusini P, Johnson CA. Staging functional damage in glaucoma: review of different classification methods. Surv Ophthalmol. 2007;52(2):156-79. doi:10.1016/j.survophthal.2006.12.008. https://doi.org/10.1016/j.survophthal.2006.12.008

12. Hodapp E, Parrish II RK, Anderson DR. Clinical decisions in glaucoma. St Louis, MO: Mosby; 1993.

13. Hood DC, Raza AS, de Moraes CG, et al. Initial arcuate defects within the central 10 degrees in glaucoma. Invest Ophthalmol Vis Sci. 2011;52(2):940-6. https://doi.org/10.1167/iovs.10-5803

Chapter 8

24-2C: a new modality of visual field analyzer

This chapter discusses the 24-2C, a new test grid and a new modality of VF analyzer that was commercially introduced on the HFA in early 2019.

1. A quick recapitulation

Early glaucomatous damage often affects the macula and damages central vision, and this damage can be among the first signs of glaucoma.[1] However, the 24-2 VF test with a 6° grid underestimates and even misses altogether central VF loss in glaucoma.[1-5]

In contrast to the 24-2 test pattern, central VF loss or macular damage in glaucoma is well documented by the 10-2 test pattern with a 2° grid with 68 points. However, a 10-2 VF test alone can miss defects identified by the 24-2 VF.[5] Adding routine 10-2 testing along with 24-2 testing to a perimetry testing regimen to detect CVFDs could be a way out. Nonetheless, performing both a 10-2 and 24-2 VF test is neither a realistic nor a feasible solution in clinical practice, especially if both eyes need to be tested.

1.1. Difficulty in replacing the 24-2 VF test

Alternative VF test patterns that more heavily sample the central retina have not been widely accepted by clinicians. Some reasons prompt clinicians not to abandon the 24-2 VF test. First, clinicians are very familiar with the 24-2 VF test and have learned how to interpret the 24-2 VF test report. Second, the 24-2 VF is ideal for detecting classic arcuate glaucomatous damage.

2. An attempt to modify the 24-2 VF test pattern

It has been studied that the inferior retina (upper VF) containing the region is vulnerable to the glaucomatous local deep defects close to fixation,[1] and testing this region with high-resolution VF data may provide more information on VF damage in this region. A schematic model has been suggested for additional points to be placed in this region to improve the ability of the 24-2 test pattern to detect macular damage. Hence, to address the issue of underestimation of glaucomatous macular damage by testing with 24-2 VF, recent research proposed modifying the 24-2 VF test by adding test point locations from the 10-2 pattern for the detection of early glaucomatous defects.[6] Specifically, the following modifications have been tried.

3. Modified VF test patterns

The 24-2 VF test pattern (6° stimulus grid) had been modified by selecting particular subsets of points from the 10-2 VF (2° grid) and adding these points to the 24-2 VF for each eye. For the stimulus locations that the 24-2 VF shares with the 10-2 VF, the TD values and probabilities from the 24-2 VF were used in the simulated VFs. Three modified 24-2 VF test patterns were simulated.[8]

3.1. 24-2 +4 VF

The first modification, the 24-2 +4 VF (Fig. 8-1A), added 4 test points, 2 in each hemifield, to create a 24-2 +4 test pattern.[7] In this modification, they added 2 additional test points from the 10-2 test pattern, located at (1°, 5°) and (-1°, 5°), to the upper hemifield of the 24-2 VF.[7] Said modification would allow the detection of relatively common and very serious arcuate defects close to fixation in the upper hemifield.[6]

3.2. 24-2 +16 (Even) VF

Another modification, the 24-2 +16 (Even) VF (Fig. 8-1B), was tried by adding 8 test points to both the upper and lower VF hemifields to improve the detection of glaucomatous macular damage.[7] This modification tested the effect of adding 16 test points selected from the 10-2 VF to further improve the ability of the 24-2 VF to detect central defects. Sixteen test points (8 per hemifield) were added so that the resulting 24-2 +16 (Even) VF test pattern

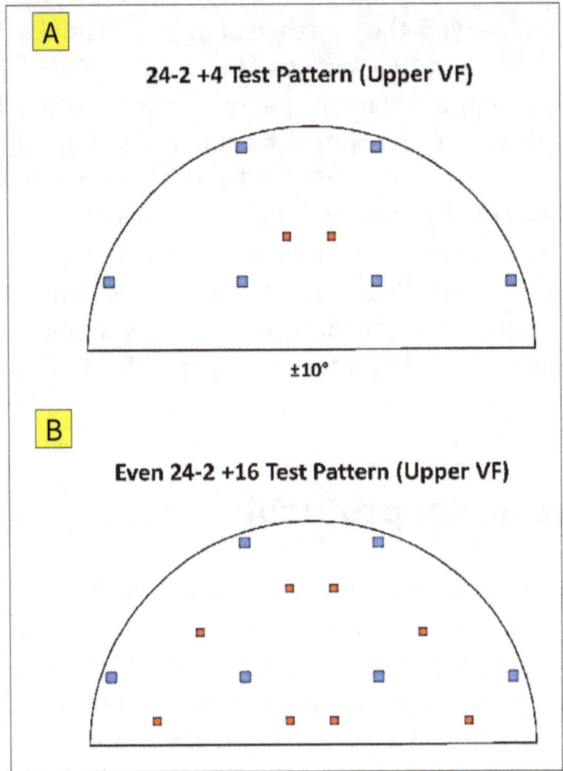

Fig. 8-1. (A) The 24-2+4 test pattern for the upper VF. It includes two 10-2 test point locations **(red squares)**. These 2 added 10-2 test points were empirically selected in an independent dataset of upper VF arcuate defects. **(B)** The test point locations of the 24-2+16 (even) VF for the upper hemifield. Eight 10-2 points per hemifield **(red squares)** were added to the 24-2 pattern to evenly sample the central 10°. In both **(A)** and **(B)**, the black semicircles mark the superior central 10°, while the larger blue squares are the original test point locations of the 24-2 VF. Reproduced from Ehrlich *et al.*[8]

would have the same number of test points as the 10-2 VF (68 test points). The time needed to perform the modified VF test should not be considerably greater than that of the 10-2 VF.

3.3. 24-2 +16 (Empirical) VF

For evaluating the importance of the particular locations of the 16 added test points, investigators simulated an empirical 24-2 +16 VF. The 16 additional points of the 24-2 +16 (Empirical) VF were chosen based on the test points that were most often abnormal with macular defects. In each hemifield, the eight test points that had the highest percentage of abnormal points were added.

Investigators observed the enhancement of sensitivity for detecting central defects by adding 10-2 test point locations to the 24-2 test pattern. For instance, by adding 8 test points per hemifield in an evenly distributed pattern, the number of true positives (for a fixed specificity of 85%) increased by 24% in the upper VF and by 17.4% in the lower VF.[7] It was found that the 24-2+4 VF performed slightly worse than the 24-2+16 (Even) VF. The real issue was how to ensure the optimal number of points to add to improve the detection of macular damage without lengthening the test time duration. Some recommended adding 16 test point locations (8 per hemifield) to the 24-2 VF test pattern to improve the detection of macular damage.[7]

4. Modified 24-2C protocol

A recently available commercial modification of the 24-2 test is the 24-2C. In 24-2C, 10 central test points from the 10-2 test grid have been added to the standard 24-2 test pattern in the central 10° (Fig. 8-2), yielding a total of 64 points, for detecting glaucomatous macular defects. These additional points, 5 in each hemifield, have been added within the central 10° of fixation. Peripheral and central VF testing can be undertaken within a single examination with a modified 24-2C protocol after the additional 10 central test points. Unlike the rest of the test grid and the 10-2, the additional points are not symmetrically distributed across the vertical or horizontal midlines in 24-2C. The locations of the added test points were derived from the most vulnerable areas of the macula (test locations commonly affected by glaucoma) to help detect damage in all stages of glaucoma. Modifications of the 24-2 where additional test locations are placed in the central VF aim to provide an alternative to conducting a full 10-2 test. Another potential practical advantage of deploying the 24-2C is that it reduces test time by around 50% from the conventionally used SITA Standard.

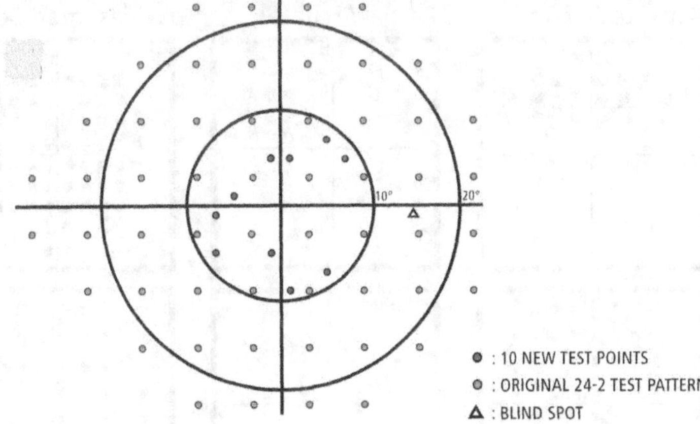

Fig. 8-2. The new 24-2C, where central test points from the 10-2 test grid have been added to the 24-2 test in the central 10° to enhance its ability to identify glaucomatous macular defects. Reproduced from Heijl and Patella.[8]

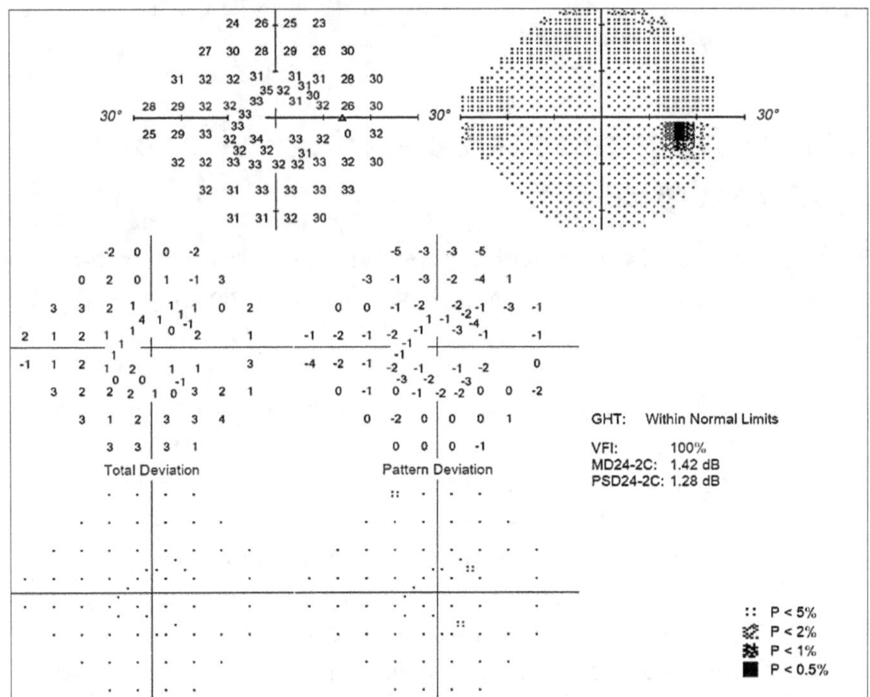

Fig. 8-3. Normal 24-2C VF: This 24-2 VF presents a normal VF without any central or peripheral field damage with GHT Within Normal Limits, VFI 100%, MD 1.42dB, and PSD 1.28 dB.

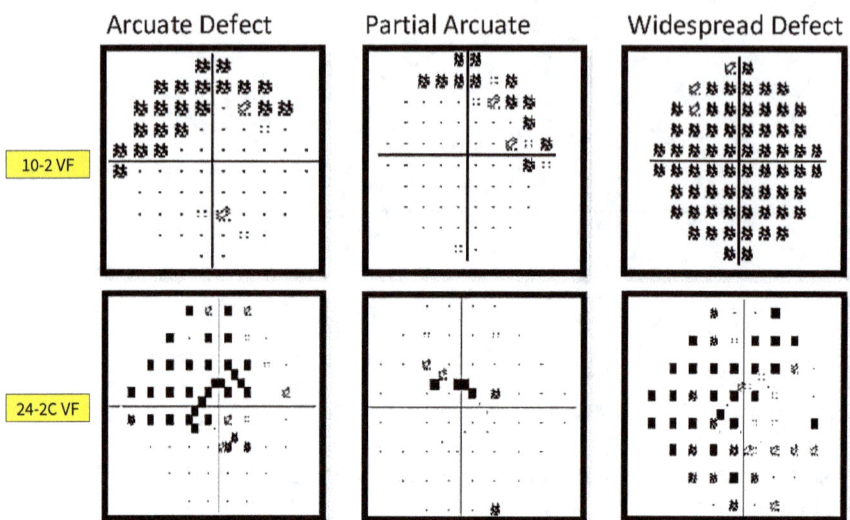

Fig. 8-4. Examples of CVFD patterns on the 10-2 **(top)** and 24-2C (bottom) testing grids. **(Right)** Arcuate defect, **(middle)** partial arcuate defect, and **(left)** widespread defect. Reproduced from Chakravarti *et al.*[9]

5. Identifying and characterizing CVFDs on the 24-2C test grid

Figure 8-3 shows a 24-2C VF without any CVFDs. CVFDs are detected when any 1 of the following pattern defects (Fig. 8-4) is identified on the 24-2C test grid:[9]

- Arcuate defect: A continuous, dense, superior or inferior hemifield defect formed by abnormal points ($P \leq 1\%$) on the TD or PD plot that includes both the nasal and temporal quadrants.
- Partial arcuate defect: A continuous superior or inferior hemifield defect formed by abnormal points ($P \leq 1\%$) on the TD or PD plot that includes both the nasal and temporal quadrants but is less dense (fewer abnormal points) than an arcuate defect.
- Widespread defect: VF sensitivity loss in all 4 quadrants of the VF on the TD or PD plot.

6. Do additional central points on 24-2 testing improve detection?

Several studies compared the efficacy of the 24-2C in detecting central defects with existing test patterns (24-2 and 10-2). Here we present the important and relevant findings as well as the concluding remarks from those studies.

6.1. The 24-2C test pattern detected fewer defects than the 10-2 test pattern

Chakravarti *et al.* compared the 10-2 and 24-2C VF tests among healthy participants (18), glaucoma suspects (12), and glaucoma patients (62).[9] Among the 62 glaucoma patients were 54 early glaucoma eyes (MD < -6 dB), 21 moderate (MD = -6 to -12 dB), and 10 advanced (MD > -12 dB) glaucoma eyes. More CVFDs were detected by the 10-2 test than by the 24-2C test in the superior and inferior hemifields. Precisely, the number of glaucoma and glaucoma suspect eyes with any CVFD from the 10-2 and 24-2C test based on TD plots was 43.9% and 31.8%, respectively. These values were almost similar based on PD plot criteria. On 10-2, the TD plots displayed the largest number of hemifield-specific CVFDs ($n = 45$) and the largest overall number of CVFDs ($n = 58$) in the superior hemifield.

The larger number of CVFDs detected with 10-2 can be explained partly by the greater number of test points on the 10-2 test grid ($n = 68$) compared with the lesser number of test points in the central 10°on the 24-2C test grid ($n = 22$) for evaluating the central 10° of the VF.

6.1.1 Agreement between the 10-2 and 24-2C VF test protocols for detecting any CVFDs based on the TD and PD criteria

Despite the greater number of CVFDs detected by the 10-2 protocol, its agreement with the 24-2C protocol for detecting any CVFDs based on the TD and PD criteria was moderate to substantial.[9] For detecting any superior CVFD, the level of agreement between the 10-2 and 24-2C tests was best on the TD plots ($k = 0.708$) and worst for detecting any inferior CVFD ($k = 0.477$). For the PD plots, agreement was best for detecting any inferior CVFD ($k = 0.689$); the agreement was less for detecting any superior CVFD ($k = 0.397$). In all of the cases, the 24-2C test pattern detected fewer defects than the 10-2 test pattern (Fig. 8-5).[9]

Agreement/Disagreement	10-2 Test Grid	24-2C Test Grid
A. Agreement: CVFD in the superior hemifield was detected by both tests.	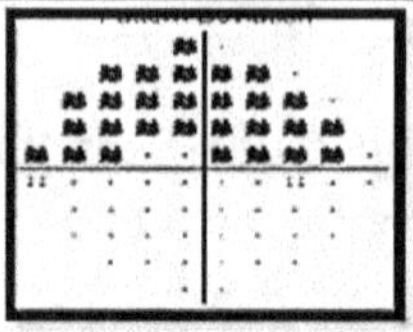	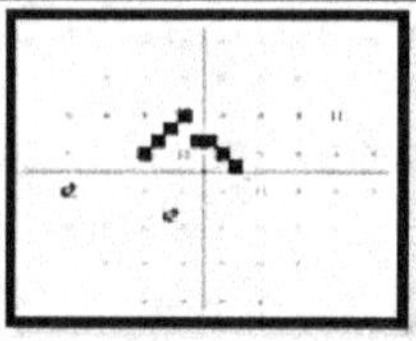
B. Agreement: CVFD in the inferior hemifield was detected by both tests	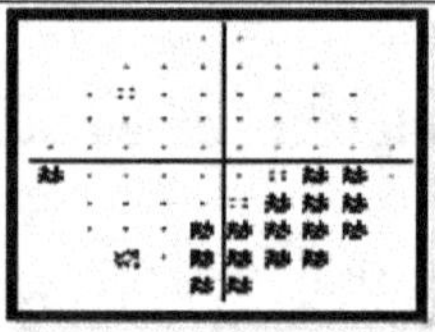	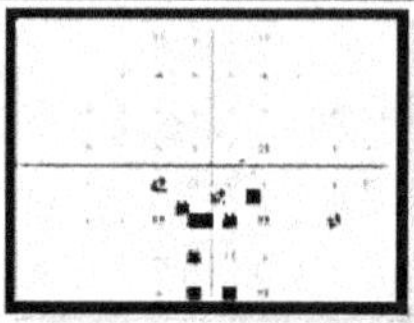
C. Disagreement: CVFD in inferior hemifield detected by 24-2C but not by 10-2.	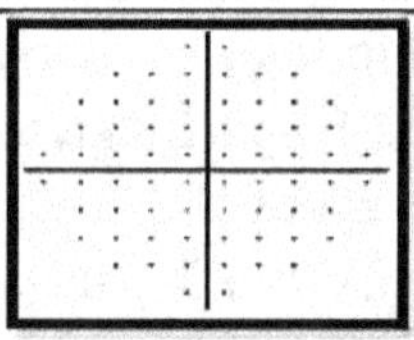	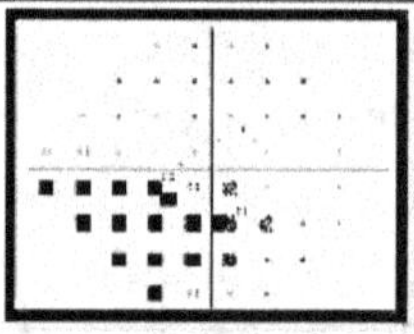
D. Disagreement: CVFD in inferior hemifield detected by 10-2 but not by 24-2C in the central 10 degrees.	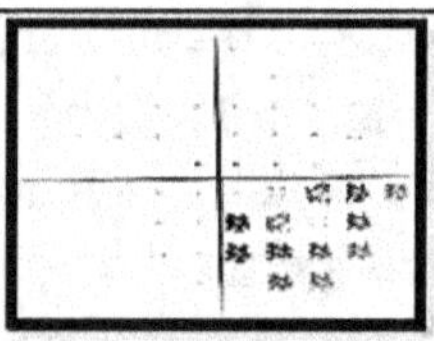	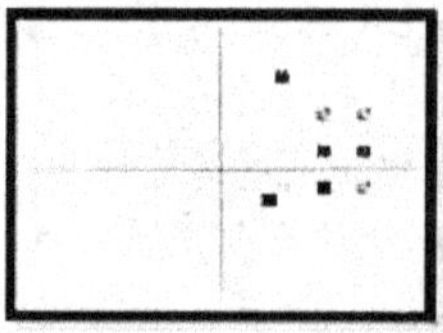
E. Disagreement: CVFD in superior hemifield detected by 10-2 but not by 24-2C in the central 10 degrees.	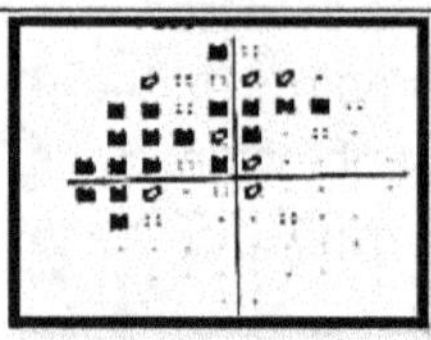	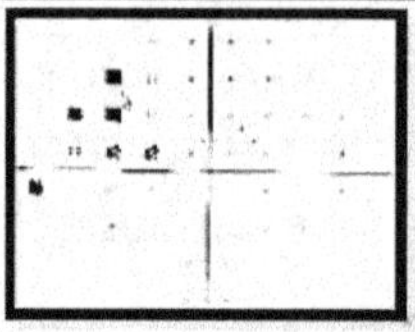

Fig. 8-5. Case examples of agreement and disagreement between the 10-2 and 24-2C tests for detecting CVFDs using the PD criterion. **(A, B)** Examples of agreement between 10-2 and 24-2C tests for the detection of a CVFD in the superior and inferior hemifield, respectively. **(C–E)** Examples of disagreement between 10-2 and 24-2C tests for the detection of a CVFD. **(C, D)** Examples of disagreement in the inferior hemifields and E shows disagreement in the superior hemifield. Note that **(D, E)** show disagreement between 10-2 and 24-2C tests for detecting **(D)** inferior and **(E)** superior CVFDs, where no CVFD is detected by the 24-2C test despite 10-2 showing distinct CVFDs. Reproduced from Chakravarti *et al.*[9]

6.2. The 24-2C detected more defective points than the 24-2 in central 10° and the 10-2 algorithm detected more defective points than the 24-2C

Behera *et al.*[10] compared the 24-2C Faster, 24-2 SITA, and 10-2 test among 60 patients with glaucoma, including 29 early glaucoma eyes (MD < -6 dB) and 31 moderate-advanced glaucoma eyes. On average, the 24-2C Faster detected more abnormal central points on the TD plot and the PD plot than the 24-2 SITA Standard in the central 10°. However, the 10-2 algorithm detected more abnormal points on the TD plot than the 24-2C Faster (2.5 times more points on the TD plot).

6.3. Both 24-2 and 24-2C test grids detect a comparable number of cluster defects for identifying central defects

Phu and Kalloniatis[11] compared the 24-2C (SITA-Faster) test with the standard 24-2 VF (SITA Standard or SITA Faster) test for detecting clusters of VF defects among 100 participants with glaucoma or glaucoma suspects. The study tested 2 cohorts of patients. In the first cohort, patients were tested on the 24-2 grid using the SITA Standard paradigm and 24-2C grid using the SITA Faster algorithm. In the second cohort, patients underwent testing on both the 24-2 and the 24-2C using SITA Faster. The aim of this study was to evaluate the clinical utility of the 24-2C. The 24-2C with an additional 10 points within the central 10° for identification of defects and correlations with structural findings has a major advantage and clinical benefit over the commonly used 24-2 test grid.

However, this study indicated that the global index results are similar to the 24-2 and 24-2C grids and both can detect a comparable number of clusters of VF defects (Fig. 8-6). Centrally, the 24-2C identifies more clusters of defects compared to the 24-2, as shown in Figure 8-6,[11] but this may not be statistically significant. The additional 10 central points in the 24-2C test only detected 2 additional cases with a cluster defect compared with the standard 24-2 grid.[11] Further evidence is needed to prove its implications on disease staging and its benefit for clinical management.

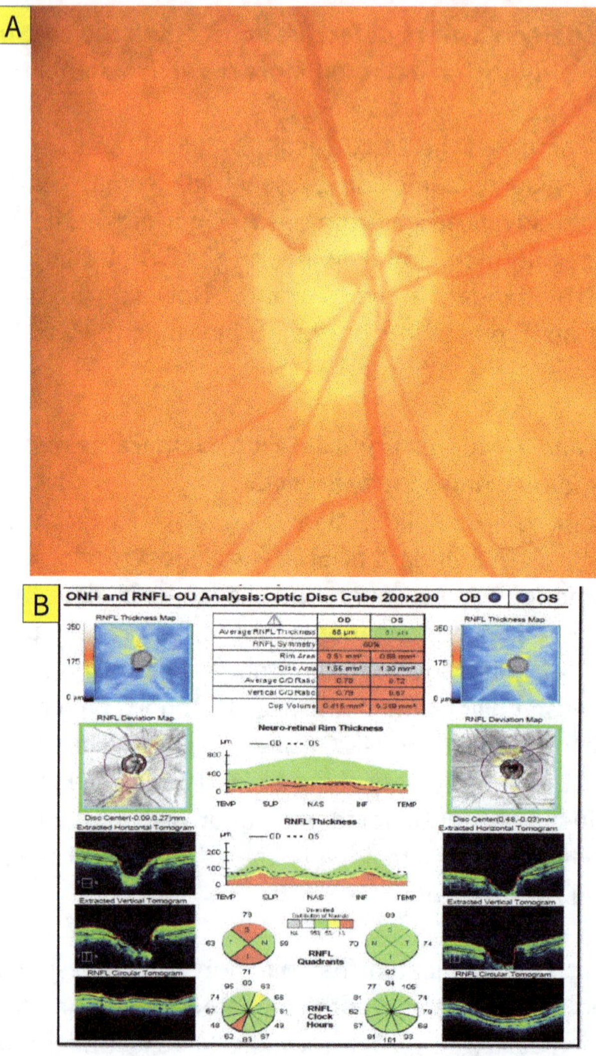

Fig. 8-6. Comparing 24-2 and 24-2C test grids for identifying glaucomatous CVFDs. **(A)** The right eye of a 68-year-old patient diagnosed with POAG. This patient presents with inferotemporal loss of neural rim in the right optic disc. **(B)** OCT confirms the presence of this impairment in both the optic nerve and RNFL. **(C)** The 24-2 VF of the patient's right eye shows a superior arcuate defect with moderate disease severity based on MD staging system (MD = -8.26 dB). The classical arcuate scotoma seen in the upper hemifield of the VF is in good agreement with optic disc findings and OCT findings shown in **(A, B)**. **(D)** His VF defect (right eye) on 24-2C agrees with the 24-2 VF and similarly shows a clear superior arcuate defect that includes the additional 10 central points from the 10-2 test pattern. Global index results are similar between the 24-2 (VFI 73%, MD -8.26 dB, PSD 11.96 dB) and 24-2C grids (VFI 74%, MD -9.03 dB, PSD 11.06 dB), and both detect almost equal numbers of clusters of VF defects. However, centrally, the 24-2C identifies more clusters of defects compared to the 24-2.

C

24-2 VF
30° 30° 30°
Total Deviation
Pattern Deviation
GHT: Outside Normal Limits
VFI: 73%
MD: -8.26 dB P < 0.5%
PSD: 11.95 dB P < 0.5%
:: P < 5%
P < 2%
P < 1%
P < 0.5%

D

24-2C VF
30° 30° 30°
Total Deviation
Pattern Deviation
GHT: Outside Normal Limits
VFI: 74%
MD24-2C: -9.03 dB P < 0.5%
PSD24-2C: 11.06 dB P < 0.5%
:: P < 5%
P < 2%
P < 1%
P < 0.5%

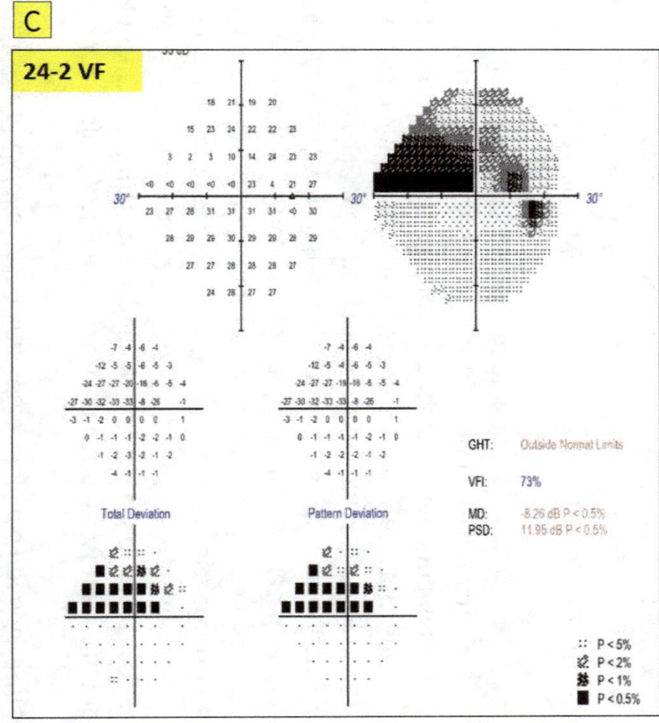

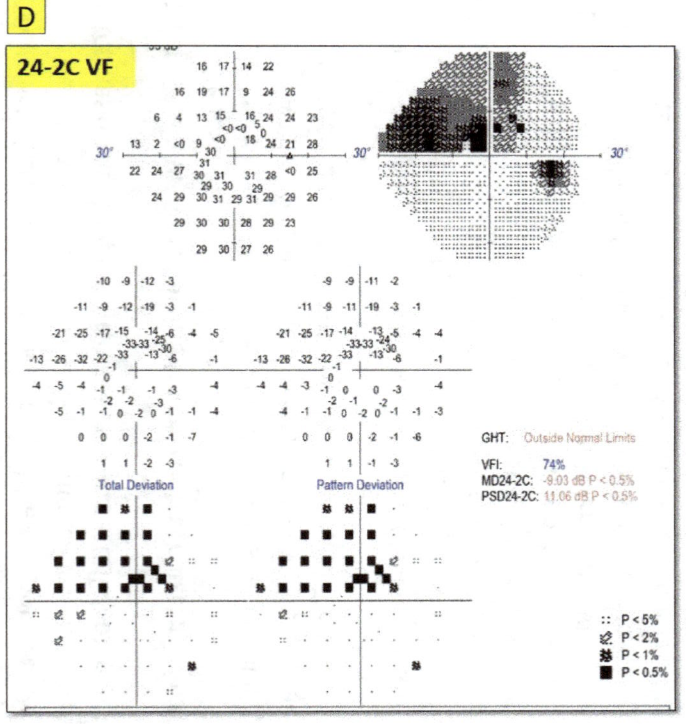

6.3.1. The additional test points in the 24-2C did not add further statistically significant clusters

For the majority of patients, the additional test points in the 24-2C did not add further statistically significant clusters (3 or more contiguous points) to identify glaucomatous CVFDs.[11] This finding indicates that, in comparison to the conventional 24-2, 24-2C does not always contribute to a criterion of cluster formation where a VF result may be considered glaucomatous. However, this particular "cluster" criterion is related to the entirety of the 24-2 test grid, which has a symmetric distribution of equally spaced (along x- and y-axes) locations, unlike the 24-2C exclusive points.[11] These observations highlight the need to revise classical glaucoma VF diagnostic CC, which may underestimate the extent of functional loss.[11] This observation on the inadequacy of the existing CC rule for detecting early glaucomatous VF loss is also discussed in Chapter 4.

6.3.2. Using 24-2C in clinical practice may not be as useful as hypothesized

Investigators expressed concern that, although the 24-2C test locations resulted in more instances of structure-function agreement compared to the 24-2, half of the test locations in the 24-2C grid did not coincide with the defects in the RGC thickness map.[11] Hence, applying 24-2C in clinical practice may not be as useful as it was thought given that currently available outcomes do not suggest an increased clinical utility of the 24-2C.

6.4. The 10-2 VF test identified more central cluster defects than the 24-2C VF test

In a separate study, Phu and Kalloniatis, compared the ability of 24-2C and 10-2 (SITA Fast) test grids to identify central VF defects and their structure-function correlation with spectral domain OCT macular imaging.[12]

A one-on-one comparison was conducted to understand the ability of the 24-2C and 10-2 test grids to identify CVFDs in a cohort of 131 glaucoma patients and 57 glaucoma suspects, and compare the global indices, test duration, point-wise sensitivity, and probability scores across the patterns in identifying and characterizing glaucomatous VF loss. Significantly more central cluster defects were identified by the 10-2 VF test than the 24-2C VF test: 31.4% identified only by the 10-2, 2.1% detected only by the 24-2C, 26.1% detected by both tests, and 40.4% detected by neither ($P < 0.0001$). The detailed findings of this study are described below.

6.3.1. Global indices: 24-2C versus 10-2

The 24-2C and 10-2 test grids yield similar global indices of VF performance and proportionally similar amounts of central VF loss. Global indices (MD, PSD, and central mean sensitivity) were similar between the 24-2C and 10-2 grids.

6.3.2. Detecting clusters: 24-2C (64 test locations) versus 10-2 (68 test locations)

The 10-2 identified more cases with central clusters of 2+ contiguous points of deficit than the 24-2C. The 24-2C in most cases identified the presence of CVFDs but not necessarily "clusters". The relatively thinner sampling of the 24-2C central locations (22 points in the central 10°) means gaps exist between test points, thus presenting a challenge for identifying contiguity between test points.[12] The advantage of the 10-2 test grid over the 24-2C seems to be related to the test density, wherein the additional points contribute to filling in gaps between test locations to produce more "clusters" of defects. Hence, additional points in the 10-2 grid produce more "clusters" of defects and a greater rate of structure-function concordance compared to the 24-2C test grid.[12]

6.3.4. Additional 10 central points within the 24-2C grid and macular scan area

In structure-function comparisons, the 10-2 VF test also had more instances of concordance (both or neither) with SD-OCT macular RGC scans than the 24-2C VF test ($P = 0.001$). Half of the 10 central points within the 24-2C grid fall outside of a 7° x 8.4° macular scan area (Fig. 8-7). On the other hand, the higher test density of the 10-2 would facilitate a greater proportion of test locations, demonstrating improved structure-function concordance for eventual correlation with functional central vision (Fig. 8-7).[12]

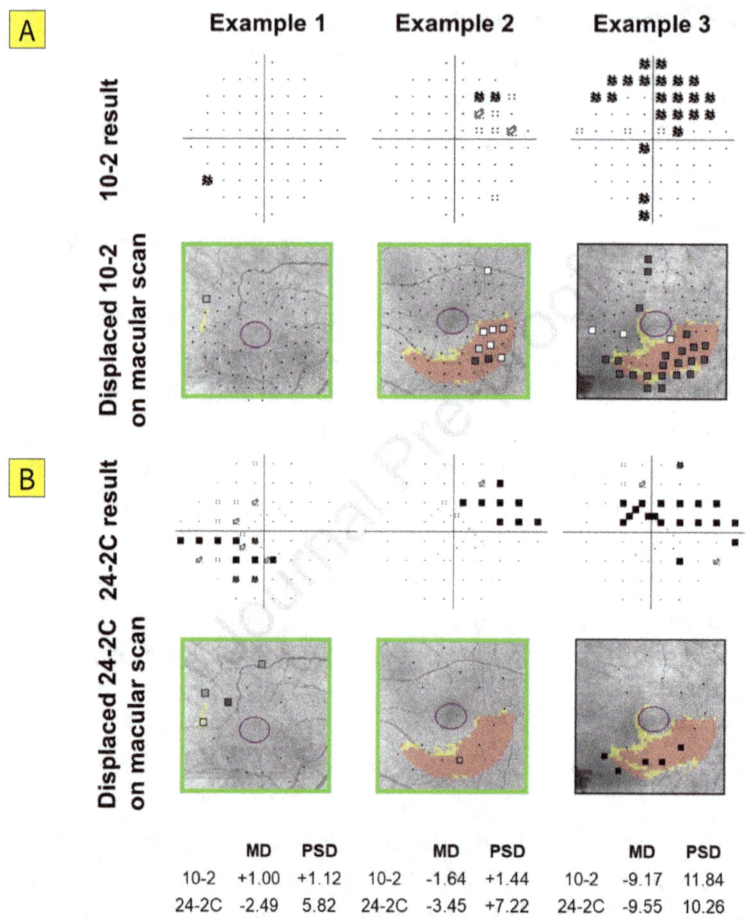

	MD	PSD		MD	PSD		MD	PSD
10-2	+1.00	+1.12	10-2	-1.64	+1.44	10-2	-9.17	11.84
24-2C	-2.49	5.82	24-2C	-3.45	+7.22	24-2C	-9.55	10.26

Fig. 8-7. Three representative examples of subjects were examined to compare the ability of the 10-2 and 24-2C test grids for identifying glaucomatous CVFDs. Each column includes (from the top to bottom rows): **(A)** the 10-2 deviation map result as per the instrument printout, the 10-2 VF test locations when shifted according to RGC displacement and flipped for anatomical comparisons with the Ganglion Cell Analysis macular scan. **(B)** The 24-2C deviation map result as per the instrument printout and the 24-2C visual field test locations when shifted according to RGC displacement and flipped for anatomical comparisons with the Ganglion Cell Analysis macular scan. MD and PSD for the 10-2 and 24-2C results are shown along the bottom row. This figure demonstrates that the 24-2C is able to detect CVFDs in manifest glaucoma and glaucoma suspect patients, but structure-function concordance and resolution of the scotoma are better by using the 10-2 test grid. Reproduced from Phu and Kalloniatis.[12]

7. The usefulness of 24-2C and 10-2

The 24-2C can identify the presence of CVFDs using similar probability criteria, while the 10-2 may be more useful in comprehensively characterizing the defects and predicting central visual function. However, the 24-2C is not as efficient as 10-2 to identify and judge the clusters. Hence a clinician should compare and assess the usefulness of the 24-2C and 10-2 for the individual patient as part of a personalized management plan. Perhaps the detection of any CVFDs on 24-2 or 24-2C could indicate conducting the 10-2 to confirm or fully characterize the central defect identified on 24-2 or 24-2C. By means of its increased test resolution, the 10-2 provides a better clarity of central vision loss. Such a comprehensive description of central vision loss is relevant for the clinician to better predict central visual function and to develop an appropriate management plan. The exact treatment plan would improve the patient's QoL and daily living activities.

8. Comparing 24-2, 10-2, and 24-2C test grids for identifying glaucomatous CVFDs in the early disease stage

Figures 8-8, 8-9, and 8-10 present 3 glaucoma cases comparing the 24-2, 10-2, and 24-2C test grids for identifying glaucomatous CVFDs in the early disease stage. In Figure 8-8, 24-2C poorly demonstrates the characteristics and severity of CVFD in comparison to 10-2 VF. In this case, while the CVFD is obvious as a deep arcuate-like PFS on the 10-2 test pattern, the 24-2C displays a partial arcuate defect in the PD probability plot. Similarly, Figure 8-9 reveals how the 24-2C VF did not detect a definite CVFD that was well recognized by the 24-2 VF and perfectly identified by the 10-2VF.

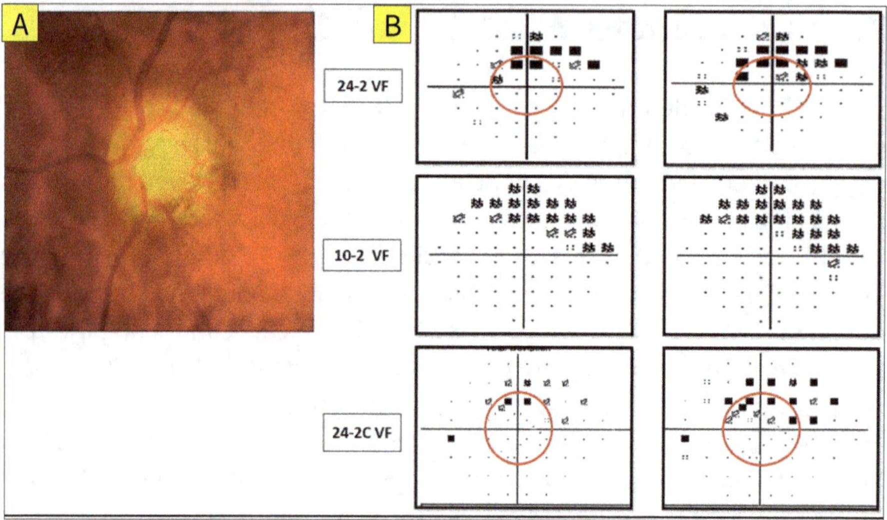

Fig. 8-8. Glaucomatous optic neuropathy and associated VF loss in the 24-2, 10-2, and 24-2C test patterns. A 73-year-old man with elevated IOP bilaterally (left eye > right eye) was advised for an optic disc evaluation and VF test in July 2021. **(A)** The left optic disc shows an obvious neuroretinal rim loss in the inferior and inferotemporal quadrant. **(B)** Corresponding VF damage is seen in both the TD and PD probability plots of all 3 test patterns (24-2, 10-2, and 24-2C). The arcuate scotoma on the 24-2 and 10-2 seen in the upper hemifield of the VF is in good agreement with the optic disc photograph. The central 12 points and 22 points are highlighted with red circles in the 24-2 and 24-2C test grids, respectively. Abnormal paracentral points are present in the TD plot of the 24-2 VF. Although there are no abnormal points in the central 5° in the TD plot, abnormal central ($P < 2\%$) and paracentral points ($P < 1\%$ and $< 0.5\%$) are present within the central 10° of the 24-2 VF in the PD plot. The CVFD is obvious as a deep arcuate-like PFS on the 10-2 test pattern, both in TD and PD probability plots. However, the characteristics and severity of the CVFDs are not very evident in the 24-2C test pattern compared to the 10-2 test pattern. The 24-2C displays a pattern defect in the central 10°, which appears like a partial-arcuate defect only in the PD probability plot.

However, in Figure 8-10, a CMVFD on the 24-2 VF is recognized well across 2 other VF test grids: 10-2 and 24-2C. In Figure 8-10, 24-2 illustrates a CMVFD where only 1 of the 4 central points within the central 5° is affected. This is marked with a circle in the threshold sensitivity plot and with a blue arrow on the PD plot on 24-2 VF. CMVFDs in the 24-2 VF are described in Chapter 2. In this figure, this CMVFD is detected by the 24-2C VF and reveals a distinct superior arcuate defect, which is encircled in the figure. This central defect is even more pronounced on the 10-2 test pattern, where it appears as a deep arcuate-like PFS, also encircled in the figure.

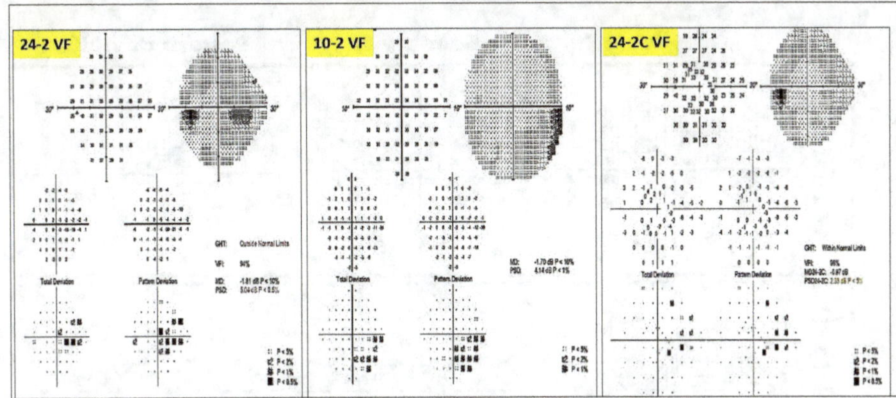

Fig. 8-9. Comparison of the 24-2, 10-2, and 24-2C test grids (PD plot) for identifying glaucomatous CVFDs in the early disease stage. This glaucoma patient in the very early disease stage presented with CVFD in the left eye. The 24-2 test grid showed abnormal central and paracentral points within the central 5° and 10°, respectively. GHT interpreted this 24-2 VF as Outside Normal Limits. Abnormal central point defects affect PSD (PSD = 5.04 dB), which is much higher than the MD (MD -1.81 dB) value. VFI is 94%. The 10-2 VF shows a clear-cut inferior arcuate-like defect (MD -1.70 dB, PSD 4.14 dB). However, the 24-2C VF fails to detect any CVFD and GHT interpretation is Within Normal Limits with 98% of VFI, MD -0.97 dB, and PSD 2.33 dB.

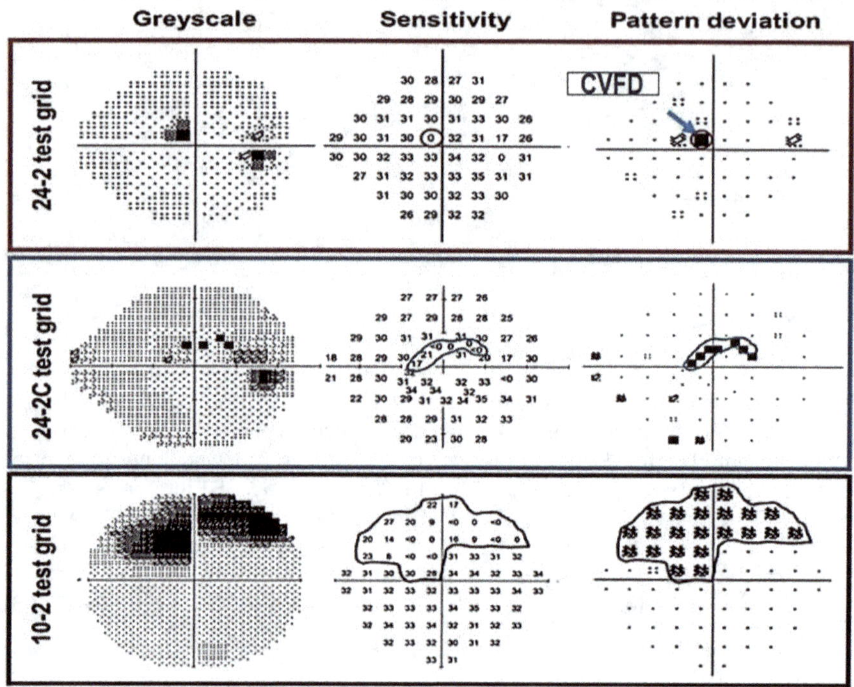

Fig. 8-10. Comparison of glaucomatous VF defects across different VF test grids. It presents the visual field test results of a 34-year-old patient with NTG who has a CMVFD on the 24-2 VF. The results demonstrate the relative outputs from 3 commonly used static perimetry test grids: the 24-2, 24-2C, and 10-2. Reproduced from Phu *et al.*[13]

References

1. Hood DC, Raza AS, de Moraes CG, et al. Glaucomatous damage of the macula. Prog Retin Eye Res. 2013;32:1-21. https://doi.org/10.1016/j.preteyeres.2012.08.003

2. Langerhorst CT, Carenini LL, Bakker D, De BieRaakman MAC. Measurements for description of very early glaucomatous field defects. In: Wall M, Heijl A, editors. Perimetry Update 1996/1997. New York, NY: Kugler Publications; 1997. p. 67-73.

3. Schiefer U, Papageorgiou E, Sample PA, et al. Spatial pattern of glaucomatous visual field loss obtained with regionally condensed stimulus arrangements. Invest Ophthalmol Vis Sci. 2010;51:5685-5689. https://doi.org/10.1167/iovs.09-5067

4. Hood DC, Raza AS, de Moraes CG, et al. Initial arcuate defects within the central 10 degrees in glaucoma. Invest Ophthalmol Vis Sci. 2011;52:940-946. https://doi.org/10.1167/iovs.10-5803

5. Traynis I, De Moraes CG, Raza AS, et al. Prevalence and nature of early glaucomatous defects in the central 10° of the visual field. JAMA Ophthalmol. 2014;132:291-297. https://doi.org/10.1001/jamaophthalmol.2013.7656

6. Hood DC, Nguyen M, Ehrlich AC, et al. A test of a model of glaucomatous damage of the macula with high-density perimetry: implications for the locations of visual field test points. Transl Vis Sci Technol. 2014;3:5. https://doi.org/10.1167/tvst.3.3.5

7. Ehrlich AC, Raza AS, Ritch R, Hood DC. Modifying the conventional visual field test pattern to improve the detection of early glaucomatous defects in the central 10°. Transl Vis Sci Technol. 2014 Dec 17;3(6):6. doi: 10.1167/tvst.3.6.6. https://doi.org/10.1167/tvst.3.6.6

8. Heijl A, Patella VM, Bengtsson B. The Field Analyzer Primer: Excellent Perimetry, 5th Edition. Carl Zeiss Meditec Inc.; 2021.

9. Chakravarti T, Moghadam M, Proudfoot JA, Weinreb RN, Bowd C, Zangwill LM. Agreement between 10-2 and 24-2C visual field test protocols for detecting glaucomatous central visual field defects. J Glaucoma. 2021;30(6). https://doi.org/10.1097/IJG.0000000000001844

10. Behera G, Nath A, Ramasamy A, Kaliaperumal S. Comparing static perimetry protocols of central field testing among patients with glaucoma. Optom Vis Sci. 2023;100(6):406-411. https://doi.org/10.1097/OPX.0000000000002020

11. Phu J, Kalloniatis M. Ability of 24-2C and 24-2 grids to identify central visual field defects and structure-function concordance in glaucoma and suspects. Am J Ophthalmol. 2020 Nov;219:317-331. https://doi.org/10.1016/j.ajo.2020.06.024

12. Phu J, Kalloniatis M. Comparison of 10-2 and 24-2C test grids for identifying central visual field defects in glaucoma and suspect patients. Ophthalmology. 2021 Oct;128(10):1405-1416. https://doi.org/10.1016/j.ophtha.2021.03.014

13. Phu J, Khuu SK, Nivison-Smith L, Kalloniatis M. Standard automated perimetry for glaucoma and diseases of the retina and visual pathways: Current and future perspectives. Prog Retin Eye Res. 2025 Jan;104:101307. https://doi.org/10.1016/j.preteyeres.2024.101307

Chapter 9

The evolution of SITA-Faster: its benefits and limitations

The latest 24-2C protocol offers the potential advantage of enabling peripheral and central VF testing within a single examination. Apart from this potential advantage, another practical advantage of deploying the 24-2C is that sensitivity measurements are driven by the SITA Faster paradigm, which reduces test time by around 53% from the conventionally used SITA Standard. This chapter describes how this SITA Faster paradigm has evolved and its potential benefits and limitations for a better understanding of test results from the 24-2C.

1. SITA Standard, SITA Fast, and SITA Faster

SITA Standard, SITA Fast, and SITA Faster are 3 primary threshold testing strategies offered by the Humphrey perimeter. SITA Standard and SITA Fast were introduced in the 1990s. They replaced the older Full Threshold and Fastpac strategies with the same or enhanced reproducibility.[1-5]

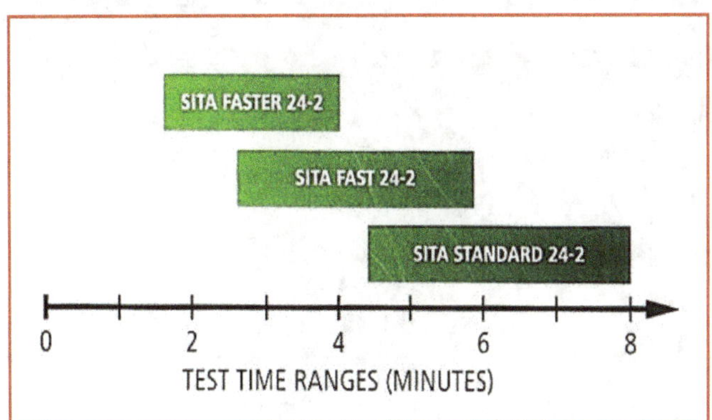

Fig. 9-1. The test times for 24-2 testing, using the three SITA strategies, in patients with glaucoma suspect and manifest glaucoma. Usually, test times increase in progressively damaged VFs. In healthy patients with normal fields, test time ranges will be shorter. Reproduced Heijl *et al.*[8]

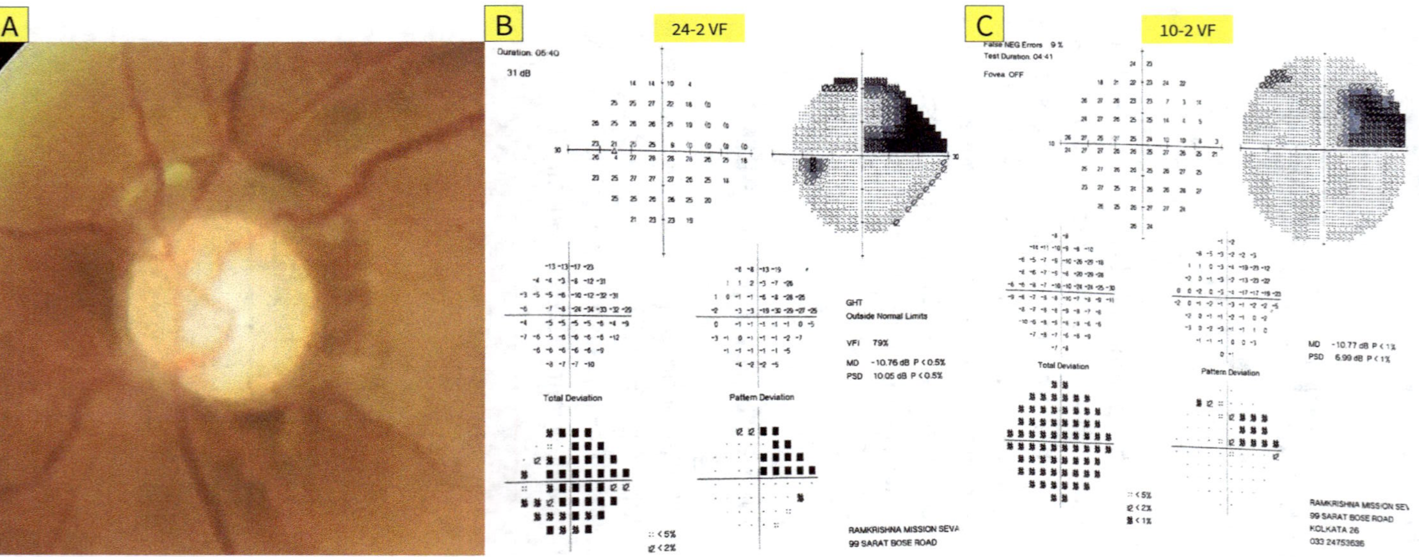

Fig. 9-2. Example of the rapid central visual field deterioration of a glaucomatous eye from an overview VF report. **(A)** A 58-year-old female patient presents with glaucomatous cupping in her left eye. The optic disc shows moderate cupping but there is a prominent inferior notch and inferotemporal nerve fiber layer defect. Absence of neuroretinal rim over less than 45° is noted. **(B)** The VF of her left eye shows a superonasal defect, more precisely an arcuate like VF defect on 24-2 VF with moderate disease severity. **(C)** She developed an early arcuate-like VF defect on 10-2 VF.

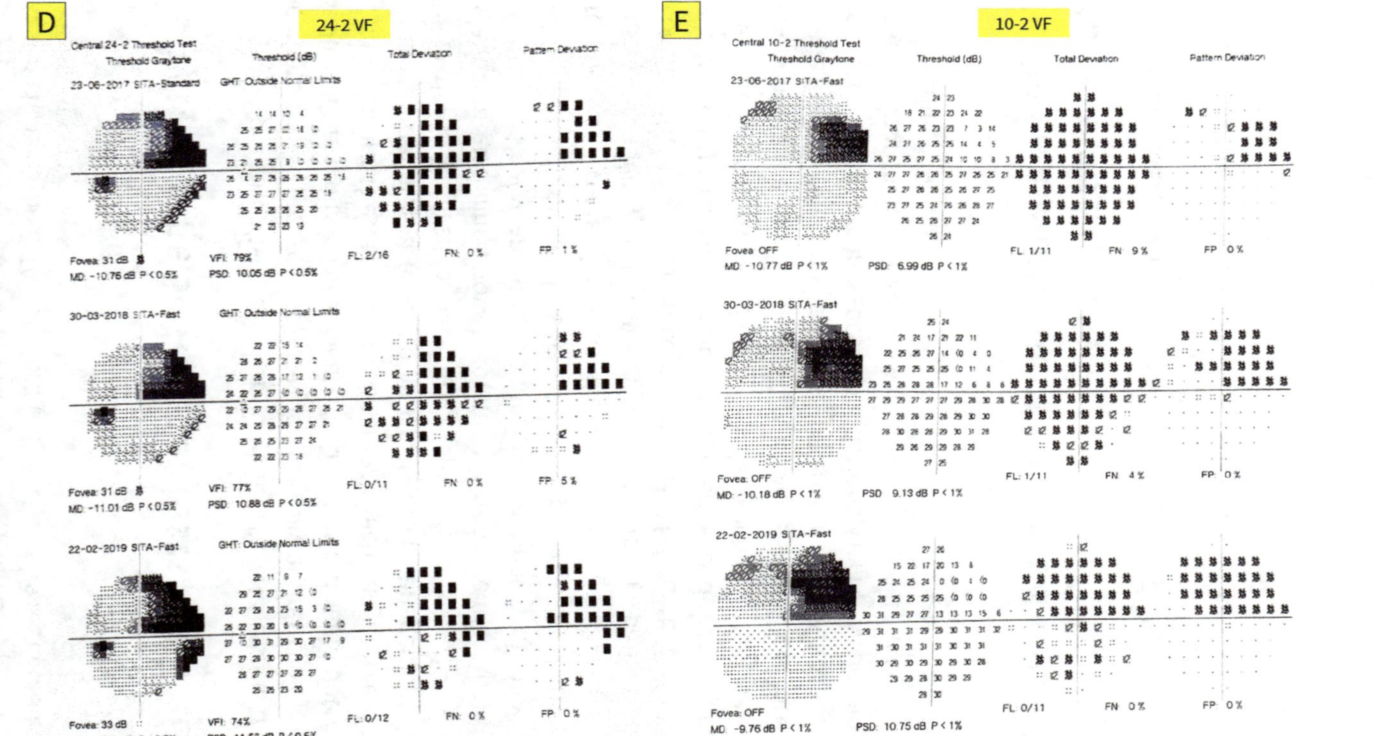

Fig. 9-2. Continued. **(D, E)** Overview reports of her 24-2 and 10-2 VF recorded her rapid worsening of central field defect and progression from 2017 to 2019. Progression was monitored with 24-2 and 10-2 VF tests. Her VFI decreased from 79% to 74% within 18 months without much change in MD or PSD values on 24-2 VF. Her progression was greater in the central field as identified with 10-2 VF. The rapid deterioration of her CVFD was reflected by a clear-cut reduction of VFI value on the 24-2VF test and progression on 10-2 VF (PSD increased from 6.99 dB to 10.75 dB on 10-2 VF) within 18 months.

The newly developed SITA Faster strategy takes approximately half the testing time of the SITA Standard (Fig. 9-1) and its repeatability is the same as that of SITA Fast.[6,7]

2. Why are the SITA Faster tests required?

A very important observation about glaucomatous eyes is that most glaucomatous eyes progress despite their IOPs always remaining within statistically normal limits.[9-11] In clinical practice, it is crucial to detect progression and measure the rate of progression, which plays a central role when setting target pressures for optimal glaucoma management. More frequent VF testing is required for detecting progression (Fig. 9-2). Therefore, several glaucoma guidelines now recommend more frequent perimetric testing in the first few years after diagnosing a patient with manifest glaucoma with glaucomatous VF loss (*e.g.*, 3 fields per year including baseline tests for the first 2 years after initial diagnosis).[12-14] In actual practice, perimetric testing frequency of newly diagnosed glaucoma patients often remains considerably lower than recommended.[15] The number of tests performed is often fewer than the number of required tests due to limited resources.[16] Hence, the alternative is to use a shorter perimetric threshold testing which could make it easier for healthcare providers to follow current glaucoma management recommendations. To encourage healthcare providers to follow current glaucoma recommendations, Heijl *et al.* developed a shorter testing algorithm, SITA Faster, which was derived from SITA Fast, to reduce the burden of testing.[17]

3. Seven modifications were made to SITA Fast to develop SITA Faster

SITA Faster has been introduced to replace SITA Fast. Anders Heijl and colleagues performed both simulations and clinical testing in developing SITA Faster and 7 modifications were made to SITA Fast to design SITA Faster.[17] Seven specific modifications are listed below:

(1) Using more efficient stimulus starting intensities: In SITA Faster, the test sequence begins at the age-corrected normal threshold level, hence reducing the number of stimulus presentations for most eyes.[17]

(2) Testing primary points once instead of twice: In older test programs, 2 staircase test sequences were performed at each primary point.[17] Only 1 staircase test reversal is required in SITA Faster.[17]

(3) Updating the VF model, incorporating information that was not available when SITA Fast was developed: SITA Faster's VF model uses the distribution of SITA Fast normal values, leading to more time-efficient testing.[17]

(4) Testing perimetrically blind points once instead of twice: In older strategies, test points where the test subject had not responded to the maximum stimulus intensity of the perimeter (0 dB/10,000 apostilb) were confirmed by presenting a second maximum intensity stimulus. This second check is not performed in SITA Faster.[17]

(5) Discontinuing routine use of false-negative catch trials: To assess test reliability, several "reliability parameters" have been used traditionally, namely: blind spot catch trials, false-negative responses, and false-positive responses. In SITA Faster, false-negative catch trials are no longer applied.[17]

(6) Using HFA's gaze tracker instead of the Heijl-Krakau blind spot method: In SITA Faster, the earlier method of checking fixation by projecting stimuli into the blind spot has been changed by the use of the HFA's gaze tracker.[17]

(7) Removing an unnecessary time delay after not-seen stimuli: In earlier SITA programs, an additional 300-ms delay is included after non-seen stimuli at the end of the response time window before the presence of a new stimulus. This extra delay is reduced in SITA Faster.[17]

4. MD, VFI, and test point differences in SITA Standard, SITA Fast, and SITA Faster

Heijl and colleagues observed that the MD index showed no statistically significant differences among the 3 test algorithms.[17] VFI was marginally and significantly lower with SITA Standard than with SITA Faster or SITA Fast, whereas the VFI values with SITA Fast and SITA Faster were the same.[17] Among the 3 test algorithms, there were also no statistically significant differences in the number of significantly depressed test points in probability plots. Though SITA Standard identified slightly and significantly more points $P <$ 1% in PSD maps, the difference between SITA Fast and SITA Faster was small for probability maps and test point significance.[17]

5. Reliability indices of SITA Faster at a glance

- **Blind spot catch trial is eliminated:** Heijl-Krakau's strategy was originally designed to monitor fixation. It has also been used as a reliability index. Blind spot catch trials can be replaced in the presence of gaze tracking.[17]
- **False-negative catch trials are abandoned:** False-negative rates depend more on VF status than on patient attentiveness. Glaucoma eyes have much higher false-negative rates than normal eyes. Such higher false-negative responses are more suggestive of glaucomatous VF loss than of patient reliability.[18,19] However, the recent findings confirm that false-negative rate estimation adds marginal value at the expense of slowing testing time.[20,21]
- **False-positive responses:** The number of false-positive responses did not differ significantly between SITA Faster and SITA Fast, while SITA Faster has statistically higher percentages of false-positive responses than SITA Standard. For more than 20 years, it has been well known that SITA Fast tests have higher false-positive numbers than SITA Standard.
- Elimination of the blind spot catch trials and false-negative catch trials may affect the translatability of the present results in some clinical practices.

6. Average test times in SITA Faster

- The average test time in SITA-Faster (Fig. 9-1) is nearly 2 minutes in eyes with early glaucomatous field loss and sometimes shorter in normal VFs.[17]
- Test time depends considerably on the stage of glaucomatous field loss, especially in eyes with advanced loss.
- In eyes with advanced VF loss and reduced VFI values, <40% the test time often takes twice as long—approximately 4 minutes for SITA Faster.[17] However, in end-stage glaucoma, it may take slightly more time.[17]
- For an earlier detection of progression and for evaluating the rate of progression, frequent testing is important.[22-24] Comparing between SITA Standard and SITA Fast in this regard,[25] this new shorter test may be preferable to increase test frequency.
- Finally, SITA Faster saves considerable test time and provides the same results as SITA Fast.

References

1. Bengtsson B, Olsson J, Heijl A, Rootzén H. A new generation of algorithms for computerized threshold perimetry, SITA. Acta Ophthalmol Scand. 1997 Aug;75(4):368-75. https://doi.org/10.1111/j.1600-0420.1997.tb00392.x

2. Bengtsson B, Heijl A. SITA Fast, a new rapid perimetric threshold test. Description of methods and evaluation in patients with manifest and suspect glaucoma. Acta Ophthalmol Scand. 1998 Aug;76(4):431-7. https://doi.org/10.1034/j.1600-0420.1998.760408.x

3. Bengtsson B, Heijl A. Evaluation of a new perimetric threshold strategy, SITA, in patients with manifest and suspect glaucoma. Acta Ophthalmol Scand. 1998 Jun;76(3):268-72. https://doi.org/10.1034/j.1600-0420.1998.760303.x

4. Artes PH, Iwase A, Ohno Y, Kitazawa Y, Chauhan BC. Properties of perimetric threshold estimates from Full Threshold, SITA Standard, and SITA Fast strategies. Invest Ophthalmol Vis Sci. 2002 Aug;43(8):2654-9.

5. Bengtsson B, Heijl A. Sensitivity to glaucomatous visual field loss in Full Threshold, SITA Standard, and SITA Fast Tests. In: M. Wall, J.M. Wild, ed. Perimetry Update 1998/99. Proceedings of the XIIIth International Perimetric Society Meeting, Gardone Riviera. The Hague: Kugler publications; 1999: 3-8

6.   Lavanya R, Riyazuddin M, Dasari S, Puttaiah NK, Venugopal JP, Pradhan ZS, et al. A comparison of the visual field parameters of SITA Faster and SITA Standard strategies in glaucoma. J Glaucoma. 2020;29(9):783-788.

7.   Phu J, Khuu SK, Agar A, Kalloniatis M. Clinical evaluation of Swedish interactive thresholding algorithm-Faster compared with Swedish interactive thresholding algorithm-Standard in normal subjects, glaucoma suspects, and patients with glaucoma. Am J Ophthalmol. 2019; 208:251-264.

8.   Heijl A, Patella VM, Bengtsson B. The Field Analyzer Primer: Excellent Perimetry, 5th Edition. Dublin, CA: Carl Zeiss Meditec; 2021.

9.   Heijl A, Bengtsson B, Hyman L, Leske MC; Early Manifest Glaucoma Trial Group. Natural history of open-angle glaucoma. Ophthalmology. 2009 Dec;116(12):2271-6. https://doi.org/10.1016/j.ophtha.2009.06.042

10.   Anderson DR, Drance SM, Schulzer M; Collaborative Normal-Tension Glaucoma Study Group. Natural history of normal-tension glaucoma. Ophthalmology. 2001 Feb;108(2):247-53. https://doi.org/10.1016/S0161-6420(00)00518-2

11.   Ahrlich KG, De Moraes CG, Teng CC, Prata TS, Tello C, Ritch R, et al. Visual field progression differences between normal-tension and exfoliative high-tension glaucoma. Invest Ophthalmol Vis Sci. 2010 Mar;51(3):1458-63. https://doi.org/10.1167/iovs.09-3806

12.   European Glaucoma Society. Terminology and guidelines for glaucoma, 4th edition - Chapter 3: Treatment principles and options supported by the EGS foundation. Br J Ophthalmol. 2017;101(6):130-95. https://doi.org/10.1136/bjophthalmol-2016-EGS-guideline.003

13.   Heijl A, Alm A, Bengtsson B, et al. The glaucoma guidelines of the Swedish Ophthalmological Society. Acta Ophthalmol Suppl (Oxf). 2012;251:1-40. https://doi.org/10.1111/j.1755-3768.2012.02415.x

14.   Chauhan BC, Garway-Heath DF, Goni FJ, et al. Practical recommendations for measuring rates of visual field change in glaucoma. Br J Ophthalmol. 2008;92(4):569-73. https://doi.org/10.1136/bjo.2007.135012

15.   Quigley HA, Friedman DS, Hahn SR. Evaluation of practice patterns for the care of open-angle glaucoma compared with claims data: the glaucoma adherence and persistency study. Ophthalmology. 2007;114(9):1599-606. https://doi.org/10.1016/j.ophtha.2007.03.042

16.   Malik R, Baker H, Russell RA, Crabb DP. A survey of attitudes of glaucoma subspecialists in England and Wales to visual field test intervals in relation to NICE guidelines. BMJ Open. 2013;3(5). https://doi.org/10.1136/bmjopen-2012-002067

17.   Heijl A, Patella VM, Chong LX, Iwase A, Leung CK, Tuulonen A, et al. A new SITA perimetric threshold testing algorithm: Construction and a multicenter clinical study. Am J Ophthalmol. 2019 Feb;198:154-65. https://doi.org/10.1016/j.ajo.2018.10.010

18. Katz J, Sommer A. Reliability indexes of automated perimetric tests. Arch Ophthalmol. 1988;106(9):1252-4. https://doi.org/10.1001/archopht.1988.01060140412043

19. Heijl A, Lindgren G, Olsson J. Reliability parameters in computerized perimetry. Presented at: 7th International Visual Field Symposium 1986; Amsterdam, The Netherlands. Available from: https://www.researchgate.net/publication/283678630_Reliability_parameters_in_computerized_perimetry. Accessed November 19, 2018.

20. Yohannan J, Wang J, Brown J, et al. Evidence-based criteria for assessment of visual field reliability. Ophthalmology. 2017;124(11):1612-20. https://doi.org/10.1016/j.ophtha.2017.04.035

21. Bengtsson B, Heijl A. False-negative responses in glaucoma perimetry: indicators of patient performance or test reliability. Invest Ophthalmol Vis Sci. 2000;41(8):2201-4. https://doi.org/10.1016/S0002-9394(00)00758-3

22. Heijl A, Alm A, Bengtsson B, et al. The glaucoma guidelines of the Swedish Ophthalmological Society. Acta Ophthalmol Suppl (Oxf). 2012;251:1-40. https://doi.org/10.1111/j.1755-3768.2012.02415.x

23. Nouri-Mahdavi K, Zarei R, Caprioli J. Influence of visual field testing frequency on detection of glaucoma progression with trend analyses. Arch Ophthalmol. 2011;129(12):1521-7. https://doi.org/10.1001/archophthalmol.2011.224

24. Wu Z, Saunders LJ, Daga FB, Diniz-Filho A, Medeiros FA. Frequency of testing to detect visual field progression derived using a longitudinal cohort of glaucoma patients. Ophthalmology. 2017;124(6):786-92. https://doi.org/10.1016/j.ophtha.2017.01.027

25. Saunders LJ, Russell RA, Crabb DP. Measurement precision in a series of visual fields acquired by the standard and fast versions of the Swedish interactive thresholding algorithm: analysis of large-scale data from clinics. JAMA Ophthalmol. 2015;133(1):74-80. https://doi.org/10.1001/jamaophthalmol.2014.4237

Chapter 10

Detection of central visual field defects with the Octopus G pattern

This book intends to familiarize the readers with the key concepts of CVFDs on SAP on HFA (Carl Zeiss Meditec, Dublin, CA, USA). However, Chapter 10 touches upon the Octopus perimeter (Haag-Streit AG, Koeniz-Berne, Switzerland) to provide a concise idea of detecting and interpreting CVFDs by the G1 program of the Octopus perimeter. The G pattern was designed to serve as a multipurpose test and it offers an excellent trade-off between test duration and accuracy.[1,2]

1. The concept of the Octopus glaucoma G1 program (the test grid)

The G1 program has 73 test locations. Among the 73 test locations, 59 test locations are in the inner 30°, which is considered the most important area for glaucoma. Again, these 59 test locations are within 26° instead of the traditional 30° area. This ensures the avoidance of scotomas caused by corrected lens edges. As the grid is denser around the center, it helps detecting paracentral scotomas. Fourteen test locations are in the peripheral and mid-peripheral area out to an eccentricity of 56°. They are more concentrated on the nasal side. This distribution is helpful for the detection of a peripheral nasal step.

1.1. The Octopus G pattern

The G pattern uses a grid of unevenly distributed 59 different test locations within the central 30° of the VF (Fig. 10-1). The test-point density is higher nasally than temporally and around the macula than in the more peripheral areas.[3] This test grid also highlights the nasal step. The Octopus G1 program presents a high density of test locations in the paracentral

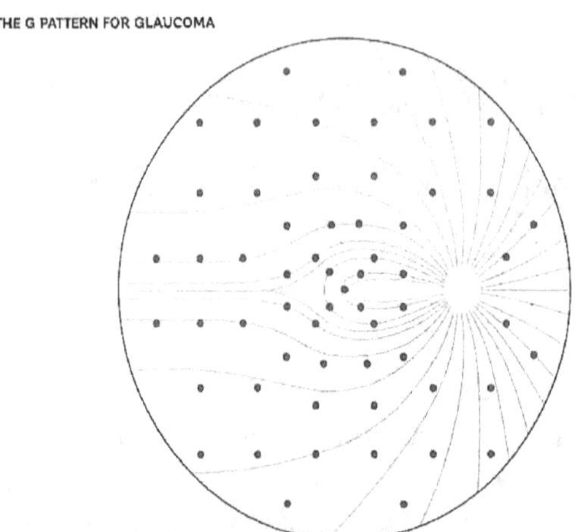

Fig. 10-1. The G pattern for glaucoma. The distribution of the test locations in the G pattern follows the retinal nerve fiber bundles. Reproduced from Racette *et al.*[3]

area (2.8° spacing) for enabling the detection of paracentral scotomas,[3] which is common in glaucoma. These paracentral scotomas are often underrated and missed by HFA 24-2/30-2.[4,5] It employs 5 central points with 2.8° separation to represent the fovea and 17 test points to test the macula.[3] This test-point distribution in G pattern allows to test the most important area of visual function for reading and object identification, and permits for additional detection of macular disease. Such test-point distribution helps both peripheral and central VF testing with increased spatial resolution in a single examination.

2. Comparing the detection rate of CVFDs between the Octopus G1 program and the 10–2 test in early glaucoma

Roberti *et al.*[6] compared the detection rate of CVFDs between the 30° Octopus G1 program (Dynamic strategy) and the HFA 10–2 SITA Standard test in eyes with early glaucoma not showing any CVFD on the HFA 24–2 SITA-Standard test. Forty-one early glaucoma patients without CVFD on the HFA 24–2 test were tested with both the HFA 10–2 test and the Octopus G1 program (Fig. 10-2).

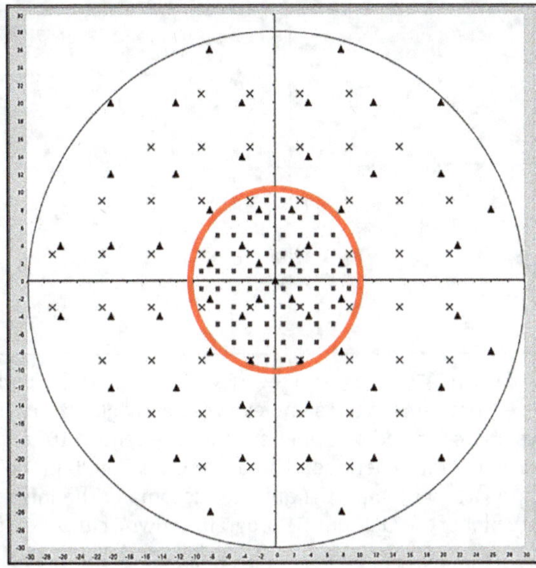

Fig. 10-2. Central 10° of the VF with the locations of HFA 24–2, HFA 10–2, and Octopus G1 plotted in the same grid. The inner circle demarcates **(red outline)** the central 10° area with test locations of the 3 tests (HFA 24–2, HFA 10–2, and Octopus G1) labeled with different symbols. Cross = HFA 24–2; square = HFA 10–2; triangle = Octopus G1. Reproduced from Roberti *et al.*[6]

The primary outcome measure was the comparison of CVFD detection rates. CVFD was defined as the presence of a cluster of 3 significantly depressed contiguous points with $P < 5\%$ on at least 2 test locations and $P < 2\%$ on at least 1 test location in the whole grid of the PD plot of the HFA 10-2 test or within the 17 central test point locations of the corrected probability plot of the Octopus G1 program. The secondary outcome measures were assessing the agreement of the test outcomes in detecting CVFDs as well as comparing test durations and the number of depressed test points outside the central 10° area between the HFA 24–2 test and the Octopus G1 program.

The HFA 10-2 test detected CVFD in 80.4% of eyes and the Octopus G1 test identified CVFDs in 56.0% of eyes ($P = 0.002$). Considering the HFA 10-2 test as the index test, the Octopus G1 program showed a sensitivity of 69.6% and a specificity of 100% for detecting a CVFD that was missed by the HFA 24-2 test. These findings demonstrated that in early glaucoma eyes where CVFDs may be missed by the HFA 24-2 test, the Octopus G1 program alone can detect CVFD with approximately 70% sensitivity and 100% specificity compared to the HFA 10-2 test (Fig. 10-3).

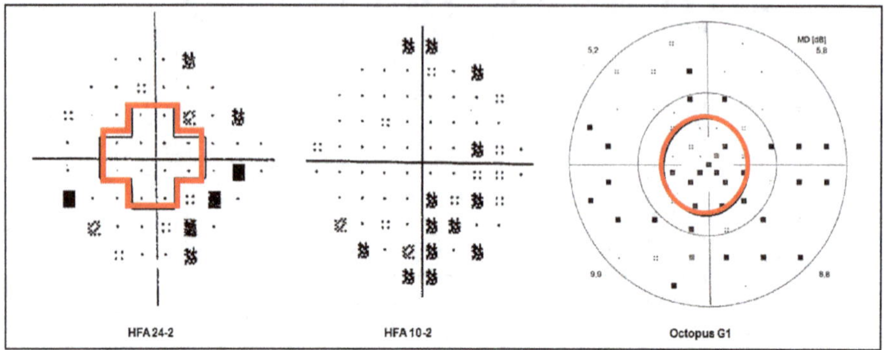

Fig. 10-3. PD plots of the HFA 24-2 test and the HFA 10-2 test, and the corrected probability plot of the Octopus G1 program of the same eye with early glaucoma. The PD plot of the HFA 24-2 test shows no depressed test points within the central 10° area **(red cross)**, but the sensitivity loss is in the more peripheral area of the VF. The PD plot of the HFA 10-2 test shows a PFS that appears to be a partial arcuate scotoma in the inferior hemifield.. The corrected probability plot of the Octopus G1 program shows a cluster of reduced sensitivity both in the central 10° area **(red circle)** and in the periphery. Reproduced from Roberti *et al.*[6]

The central VF area can be selectively and more precisely tested using the HFA 10-2 test, which uses a test-point grid of higher spatial resolution for the evaluation of the central 10° VF area. However, the HFA 10-2 test does not detect peripheral VF defects outside the central 10° area and both the 10–2 and the 24–2 tests should be performed for optimal decision-making to diagnose and manage glaucoma patients. The high specificity of the Octopus G1 program ensures a minimum of false-positive cases for CVFD detection in routine clinical practice. Hence, some investigators recommend that the Octopus G1 program may be an alternative to performing combined 24-2 and 10-2 VF tests to detect central and peripheral defects.[6]

3. Better performance of the Octopus G1 program over the HFA 24–2 in detecting CVFD

The aforementioned study indicated that the Octopus G1 program had 69.6% sensitivity and 100% specificity for detecting CVFDs.[6] The reason behind the superior performance of the Octopus G1 program over the HFA 24–2 test is that the G1 program uses 59 test point locations for the total 30° tested area, of which an increased density grid of 17 test point locations is within the macular area. On the other hand, the HFA 24-2 uses 54 test point locations for a 24° VF area, and only 12 of the 54 test points are located in the central 10°; of these, 4 locations cover the central 8° area. Again, a higher sensitivity of the HFA 10-2 test over the Octopus G1 test in CVFD detection is predictable as the HFA 10-2 test employs a test-point grid of high spatial resolution due to its 68 test point locations in the central 10°.

4. Optimal placement of stimuli for detecting CVFD with high-density perimetry

Hood and colleagues[4] proposed a model for identifying CVFDs by using high-density perimetry. The purpose of this research was to use high-density perimetry to test a model of glaucomatous macular damage (CVFD) and evaluating the optimal placement of stimuli applied for detecting central damage.

Thirty-one eyes from 31 patients were selected with the single criterion of having defects within the central 10° of the superior VF. VF testing was performed with a customized, upper hemifield VF test (Octopus 900; Haag-Streit, Inc., Koeniz-Berne, Switzerland) with double the density (diagonal spacing of 1.4°) of the 10-2 pattern.[4]

Two additional points were included to the 24-2 test pattern to have the same number of points (9) in the central 10° of the upper VF as the G1 program (Fig. 10-4).[4] This modification was done to detect glaucomatous defects and compare the ability of the grids (HFA 24-2, Octopus G, and HFA 24–2+2 test locations) to detect the average number of abnormal test points with sensitivity ≤ -5 dB.[4] To decide the optimal locations of these 2 additional points, the program tested all possible locations to maximize the average number of abnormal test points (TD ≤ -5 dB) across patients. The possible sites of additional points were restricted to a subset shared by the 10-2 VF test pattern. They observed that the Octopus G1 program performed better than the HFA 24–2 test, but the pattern in which 2 points were added to the HFA 24–2 test at -1°, 5° and 1°, 5° positions performed better than the G1 program.

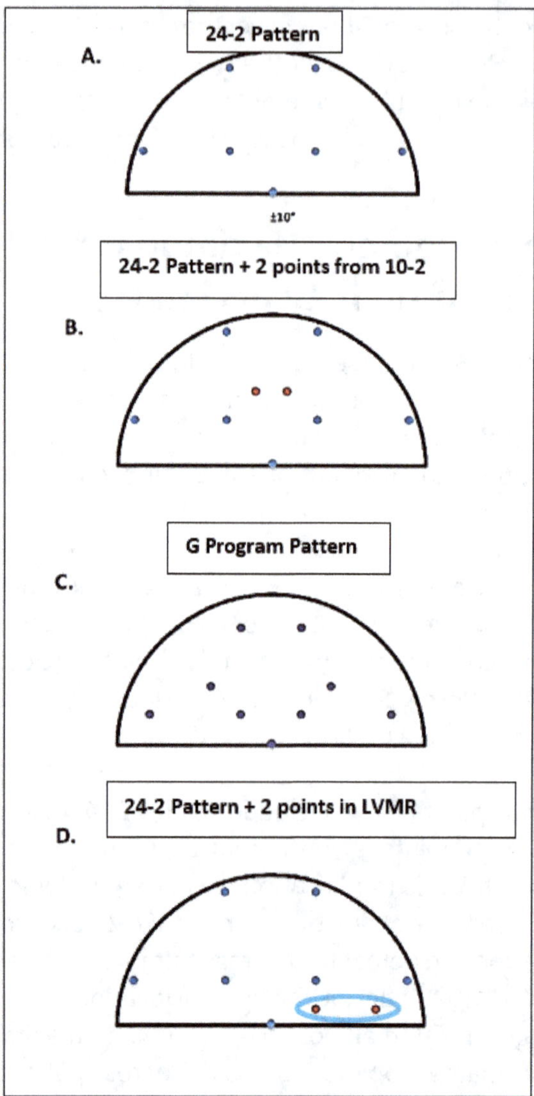

Fig. 10-4. The simulated 4 VF test patterns. **(A)** The 24-2 locations **(blue)**. **(B)** The 24-2 points **(blue)** with 2 points **(red)** added to maximize the number of points ≤ - 5 dB. **(C)** The G program has the same number of points as in **(B)**, but in different locations **(purple)**. **(D)** The 24-2 points **(blue)** with 2 points **(red)** added in the less vulnerable macular region (LVMR). Reproduced from Hood *et al.*[4]

5. Detecting central and peripheral glaucomatous VF defects simultaneously

In recent years, a plethora of researchers have felt the need for better testing of the central macular area by increasing the ability of the HFA tests to detect defects within the central 10°. Nonetheless, detecting CVFDs in routine clinical practice by performing selective macular testing demands extra time and cost. Considering this, using one test that evaluates both the central 10° area and the total 30° VF for detecting glaucomatous defects offers a useful tool. The existing Octopus G1 program pattern and Dynamic strategy are widely used instruments that together provide the benefit of detecting central and peripheral glaucomatous VF defects simultaneously. According to some researchers, it is better to consider this test for primary VF investigation in glaucoma detection until more sensitive combined central and peripheral VF tests are available.[6]

References

1. Sugimoto K, Schötzau A, Bergamin O, Zulauf M. Optimizing distribution and number of test locations in perimetry. Graefes Arch Clin Exp Ophthalmol. 1998 Feb;236(2):103-8. https://doi.org/10.1007/s004170050049

2. Messmer C, Flammer J. Octopus program G1X. Ophthalmologica. 1991;203(4):184-8. https://doi.org/10.1159/000310250

3. Racette L, Fischer M, Bebie H, Holló G, Johnson CA, Matsumoto C. Visual field digest. A guide to perimetry and the Octopus perimeter. 6th ed. Koniz: Haag-Streit AG; 2016.

4. Hood DC, Nguyen M, Ehrlich AC, et al. A test of a model of glaucomatous damage of the macula with high-density perimetry: implications for the locations of visual field test points. Transl Vis Sci Technol. 2014 Jun 19;3(3):5. https://doi.org/10.1167/tvst.3.3.5

5. Ehrlich AC, Raza AS, Ritch R, Hood DC. Modifying the conventional visual field test pattern to improve the detection of early glaucomatous defects in the central 10°. Transl Vis Sci Technol. 2014 Dec 17;3(6):6. https://doi.org/10.1167/tvst.3.6.6

6. Roberti G, Manni G, Riva I, Holló G, et al. Detection of central visual field defects in early glaucomatous eyes: comparison of Humphrey and Octopus perimetry. PLoS One. 2017 Oct 24;12(10) https://doi.org/10.1371/journal.pone.0186793

Chapter 11

Central visual field defects in advanced glaucoma

Preservation of the central VF and visual acuity is the ultimate goal of glaucoma treatment, especially in the advanced stages of the disease. In the advanced stage of glaucoma, VF loss can be defined by a field constricted to a 10° radius or less. This chapter describes CVFDs in advanced glaucoma and also highlights the implications of the 10-2 VF test for detecting the characteristics and quantifying the progression and the severity of advanced glaucoma.

1. Different terminologies to express the severity in late stage of glaucoma

There is a discrepancy in the classification systems for grading the severity of glaucoma in the late stage and different terminologies have been used. This chapter uses the term "advanced glaucoma" to encompass all terminologies (advanced glaucoma, severe glaucoma, end-stage glaucoma) commonly applied to refer to the severity of glaucoma disease in its late stage. Different terminologies and grading systems for defining the severity of glaucoma in the late stage are described below.

1.1. Definition by US Social Security Administration

According to the US Social Security Administration, eyes with VF mean deviation (MD) of -22 dB or less on 30-2 VF testing are classified as legally blind.[1] In clinical practice, glaucomatous visual loss is often assessed by the 24-2 test pattern instead of the 30-2 test pattern. So, the definition of legal blindness has often been related to the 24-2 test.[2,3] Hence, a 24-2 VF MD of -22 dB has been accepted as the cut-off point for end-stage glaucoma.

1.2. Staging system proposed by Mills *et al.*

The staging system by Mills *et al.*[4] is comprised of 6 ordered stages from Stage 0 to Stage 5 and is based on the Humphrey VF. For grading glaucoma severity, this staging system identified Stage 3, advanced glaucoma, with an MD value from -12.01 dB to -20.00 dB. For Stage 4, classified as severe glaucoma, the MD score cut-off value is -20.01 dB or worse. This grading system introduced Stage 5 as "end-stage glaucoma", a new staging for disease severity. "End-stage glaucoma" typifies eyes without any VF in the worst eye or no VF attributable to central scotoma.

1.3. Modified staging system proposed by Mills *et al.*

For grading severity, Mills *et al.* proposed altogether four stages.[5] Of these 4 stages, this classification proposed 2 stages for classifying the severity in the late stage of glaucoma, namely, the advanced stage (-12.01 dB to -22.00 dB) and severe stage (-22.01 dB or worse). This classification system does not mention any end-stage glaucoma for categorizing further worse cases.

1.4. Definition based on a recent study

For some authors,[6] eyes with MD > -15 dB on a 24-2 VF are defined and categorized as advanced glaucoma.

1.5. Staging by Treatment of Advanced Glaucoma Study

In the Treatment of Advanced Glaucoma Study (TAGS),[7] the term "advanced disease" is classified according to the Hoddap-Parrish-Anderson (HPA) classification of glaucoma severity.[8] As per the HPA classification, severe glaucomatous VF loss in 1 or both eyes at presentation is based on any of these criteria on 24-2VF:

1. MD > -12 dB.
2. More than 50% of the points (37) are depressed below the 5% level or more than 20 points are depressed below the 1% level on the PD plot.
3. At least 1 point in the central 5° has a sensitivity of 0 dB.
4. Points within the central 5° of fixation with a sensitivity of < 15 dB in both hemifields.

1.6. MD of -20 dB or lower as a severe stage of glaucomatous VF damage
A group of clinicians considers an MD of -20 dB or lower to be a severe stage of glaucomatous VF damage and such eyes are generally assumed to be close to the end stage of the disease.[9] The decision to consider a 10-2 SITA Standard VF with an MD of ≤ -15 dB as indicative of severe glaucoma damage was arbitrary and based on some clinicians' personal experience and observation.

In summary, there is no consensus on classifying the late stages of glaucoma and terminologies differ. It is important to note that the HPA system has been widely used by clinicians and for research purposes and is different from the gradings mentioned above.

2. Evaluating advanced glaucoma

An estimated 10% to 39% of patients present with advanced open-angle glaucoma (OAG), and many of them have no signs or symptoms of disease at the time of diagnosis.[10-12] Again, as the population ages with increasing life expectancy, a larger proportion of patients will develop advanced disease. These advanced glaucoma patients are at the maximum risk of becoming functionally impaired due to the severity of the disease. They also bear the burden of more expensive treatment.[13-16] Clinicians should determine whether the patient is stable on their current therapy or whether they are progressing and treatment should be intensified.

There are currently no accepted standard guidelines for which tests are most effective for detecting progression in advanced glaucoma. Using standard structural and functional testing for monitoring advanced glaucoma is extremely difficult for the clinician since both standard structural and functional tests that usually guide treatment decisions are of limited value in an advanced stage. It is harder to detect changes in eyes at an advanced stage of glaucoma with standard structural measures as the RNFL becomes quite thin, or very little of the neuroretinal rim remains.

Again, VF test points are more variable in advanced disease.[17] The global cpRNFL thickness approaches an asymptote when the MD of the 24-2 VF is approximately > -15 dB.[18,19] Hence, imaging in advanced glaucoma

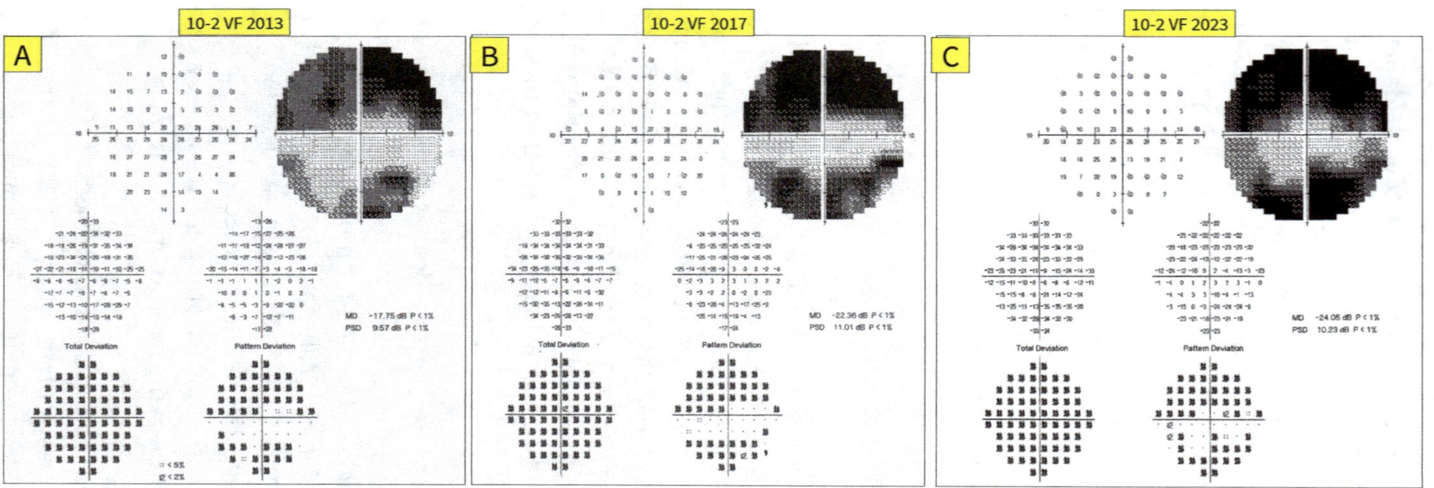

Fig. 11-1. VF findings of a 60-year-old male diagnosed as POAG who had undergone filtration surgeries in both eyes nearly a decade ago. He is blind in his left eye and his right eye (best-corrected visual acuity 20/63, logMAR +0.5) has advanced glaucoma with MD -17.75 dB on the first 10-2 VF in **(A)** (2013), followed up by 2 more 10-2 VF tests in **(B)** 2017 and **(C)** 2023. IOP was 8 mmHg in the right eye on medical therapy. His central VF loss on 10-2 VF is present in a more vulnerable, superonasal region, preserving the main less vulnerable zone.

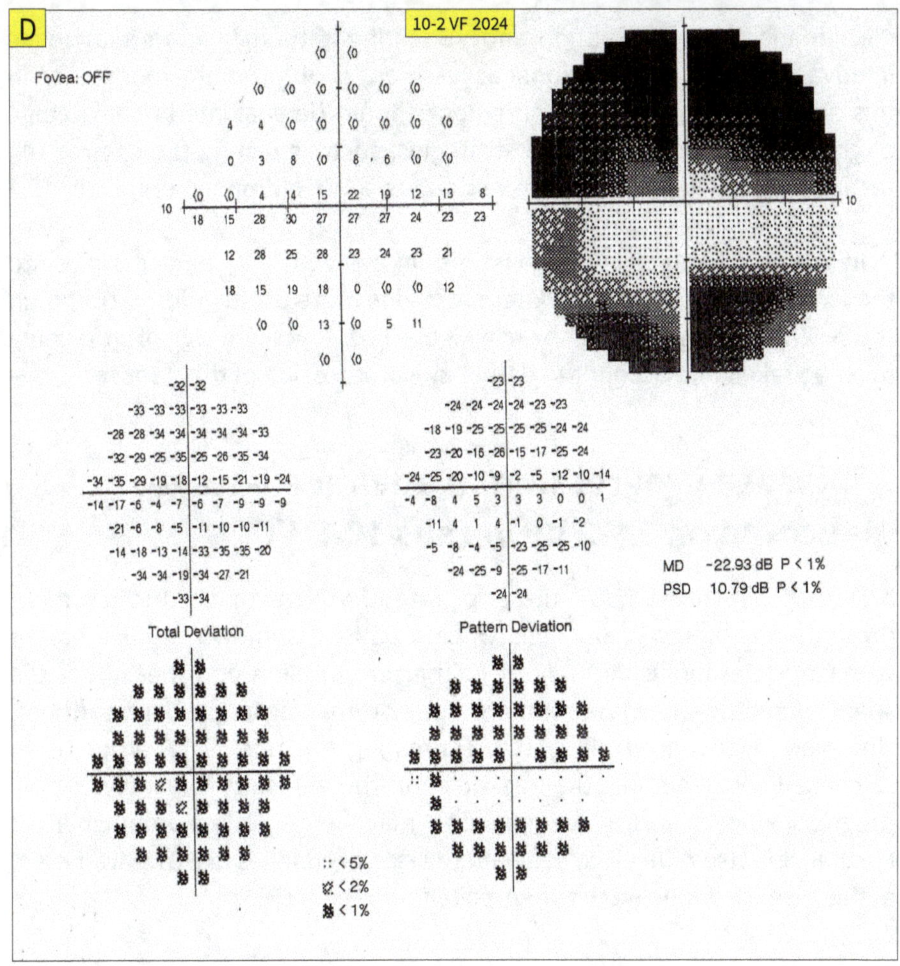

Fig. 11-1. Continued. **(D)** His central VF loss on 10-2 VF, in September 2024, shows minimal changes.

gives inadequate information and VF testing is thought more diagnostic in advanced disease. Functional assessment is of foremost importance in this advanced stage. VF measurement should be evaluated at this stage of glaucoma by using targeted strategies, such as testing the central 10°, testing a 24-2 VF field with a size V stimulus, and Goldmann perimetry.

In advanced-stage glaucoma where an eye with a VF defect is close to the fixation, the central 10° VF test provides more useful information than the 30-2/24-2 program, as shown in Figure 11-1. Any slight sign of worsening must be taken into account to detect any progression of the disease.

3. Disease progression in advanced-stage glaucoma on 24-2 VF versus 10-2 VF

It may be difficult to know the prior rate of VF loss that led to a patient presenting with severe damage. Once a patient is known to have severe damage, determining the risk of further progression and measuring the speed of deterioration is essential in decision-making for proper treatment. However, in advanced glaucoma, estimating the rate of VF progression is challenging.[20] Among the reasons for the difficulty of analyzing VF progression in severe glaucoma, one may be its low reproducibility.[21] Further, it is also difficult to evaluate the rate of changes in OCT parameters at this disease state due to the so-called floor effect.[22]

Rao *et al.* evaluated the rate of MD change in glaucomatous eyes with VF defects on 24-2 and 10-2 VF testing and underscored the importance of following up glaucoma patients, especially those with advanced VF loss, with 10-2 VFs when the central points on the 24-2 VF are affected.[23] The study observed that the rate of MD change was similar on 24-2 and 10-2 VFs in eyes with early and moderate glaucomatous VF loss, while the rate of MD change was significantly greater on 10-2 compared to 24-2 VFs in eyes with advanced glaucoma (Table 11-1). They concluded that evaluating the rate of MD change on 10-2 VFs —in patients with VF defects both on 24-2 and 10-2 VFs— is conducive to a better assessment of glaucoma progression, especially in eyes with advanced glaucoma.

In a retrospective study, Park *et al.* compared the performance of the 10-2 versus 24-2 VFs (VFs) in detecting the progression of IPFS in glaucomatous eyes.[24] They observed that in glaucoma patients with IPFS (early glaucoma), the 10-2 VF detects more progression (-0.40 ± 0.51 dB/year) compared to the 24-2 VF (-0.23 ± 0.28 dB/year).[24] They suggest that follow-up of the central VF damage in eyes with PFS is needed by using algorithms with densely spaced grids. This study has already been discussed in previous chapters.

The difference in results between the study by Rao *et al.*[23] and the study by Park *et al.*[24] may be explained by the differences in their respective inclusion criteria. Rao *et al.* included eyes where the VF defect on the 24-2 VF involved 1 of the 4 central points with a correlating affected defect on the 10-2 VF, whereas Park *et al.* investigated eyes with a strictly defined PFS with no points outside the central 10° involved on 24-2 VF.

Table 11-1. The median rate of MD change (interquartile ranges in parentheses) in different severities of glaucoma on 24–2 and 10–2 VFs at baseline

Severity of glaucoma	MD change on 24-2 VF	MD change on 10-2 VF	*P* value
MD > -6 dB (*n* = 24)	-0.40 (-0.56, -0.18)	-0.45 (-0.55, -0.28)	0.42
MD between -6 and -12 dB (*n* = 27)	-0.40 (-0.68, -0.18)	-0.32(-0.47, -0.17)	0.26
MD between -12 and -20 dB (*n* = 48)	-0.21 (-0.46, -0.06)	-0.28 (-0.51, -0.14)	0.04
MD <-20 dB (*n* = 68)	-0.06 (-0.16, 0.05)	-0.18 (-0.32, -0.05)	<0.001

Table reproduced from Rao *et al.*[23]

4. Quantifying VF progression in severe glaucoma is challenging due to the floor effect

Judging progression in patients with severe disease is particularly challenging because of the increased variability of VF defects and reduced measurable remaining visual function. Trend analyses of global indices such as MD and VFI are among the most commonly used methods for estimating the rates of VF progression (slopes).[25,26] Using MD values to quantify VF loss has limitations as it is affected by media opacities as well as other causes of generalized depression and is not specific to glaucoma. In cases of stable MD, there is less likelihood of imminent risk of visual impairment.

A study estimated the association between the severity of VF damage at presentation and the rate of VF progression in glaucoma. They found a significant positive relationship between MD and rate of progression in mild glaucomatous loss and a negative relationship in the severe glaucomatous VF loss category.[27] The study observed that the relation between MD and rate of progression was not significant in the moderate VF loss category. In advanced stages of the disease, as damage increases, the rate of progression becomes smaller; this is known as the "floor effect".[26] Therefore, trend analysis is not appropriate for detecting progression in patients with severe disease. Dissimilar criteria have been used to establish progression in glaucoma and the best method is yet to be found.

In a study on severe glaucoma, investigators observed that the number of undetectable locations increased as MD decreased (worsened), and more than 50% of the test locations had remained undetected in baseline tests.[21,28] According to this study, the lower rate of MD slopes in severe glaucoma can be accounted for by the presence of consistently undetectable test locations. Undetectable test locations appear as non-progressive locations. This also suggests that trend analyses of conventional global indices may not be ideal for estimating the rate of VF progression due to the influence of test points without detectable sensitivity (blind locations). Findings from previous research are consistent with these results, showing the undetectable reproducibility of a large number of test locations in advanced glaucoma.[9] Rao *et al.* also reported that the rate of change in the VFI becomes slower in a very advanced stage due to the floor effect and emphasized the necessity of developing an alternative for quantifying VF progression in advanced-stage glaucoma.[23] This happens because most of the peripheral points have likely reached their "floor" in these eyes with advanced glaucoma and severe VF loss. The inability to detect a further change in these peripheral points would mask the change happening in the central points when the MD is estimated by averaging the sensitivity loss across all points on a 24-2 VF. With only a central island of field remaining in these eyes, it is possible that the change would stand out better when the central VF is evaluated with greater resolution.

5. The characterization and classification of central VF loss in advanced glaucoma

Conserving the central VF is crucial for the QoL of patients with advanced glaucoma for which functionality largely depends on residual temporal vision. Hence, a better understanding of patterns of CVFDs and their development over time is of great significance in improving the management of advanced glaucoma.

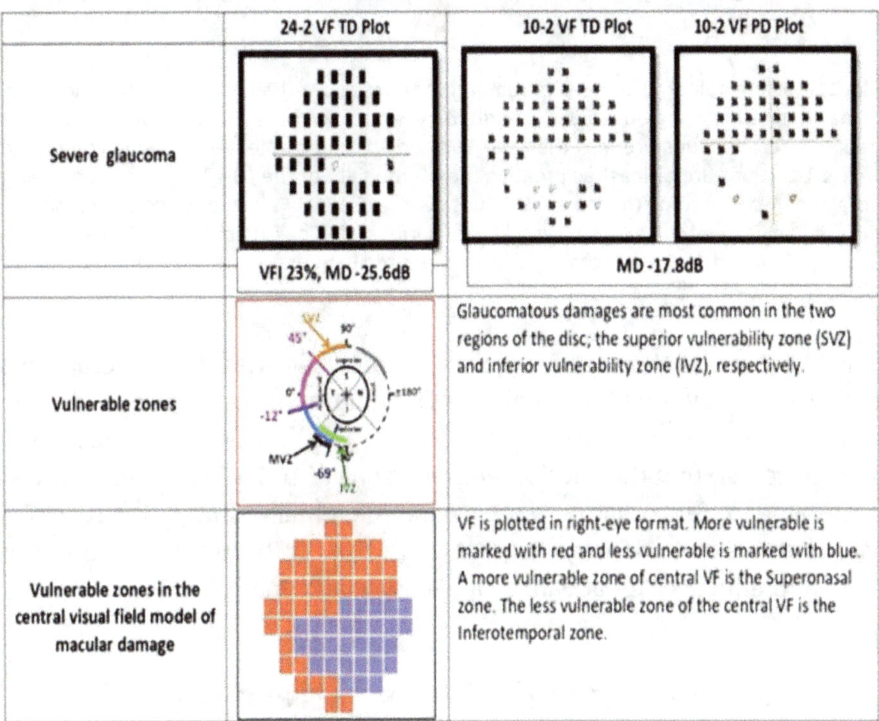

Fig. 11-2. (**Top row**) An eye with advanced glaucomatous VF loss in the right eye on 24-2 VF (PD plot) with VFI 23% and MD -25.6 dB. This advanced loss is also evident in the 10-2 VF (both TD and PD plots). The 24-2 and 10-2 VF show the patient's intact central inferotemporal region of the VF, which is less vulnerable to damage. (**Middle row**) The regions of the optic disc are most vulnerable to local glaucomatous damage. Reproduced from Hood.[30] (**Last row**) Vulnerable zones in the central VF model of macular damage in a 10-2 VF. A more vulnerable zone (**red**) of the central VF is the superonasal zone. The less vulnerable zone (**blue**) of the central VF is the inferotemporal zone. VF is plotted in right-eye format. Reproduced from Wang *et al.*[31]

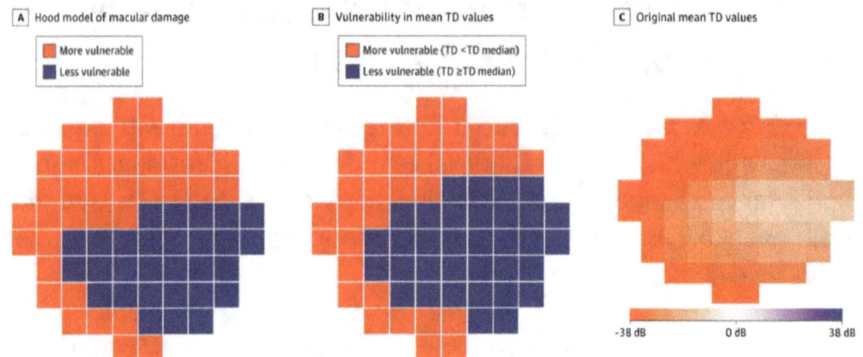

Fig. 11-3. More vulnerable and less vulnerable zones of the 10-2 central VF. **(A)** The model of macular damage in glaucoma is described by Hood *et al.*[29] **(B)** The more vulnerable zone (red: where TD values are less than the TD median) and the less vulnerable zone (blue: where TD values are at least as great as the TD median) of the 10-2 VF. These zones were obtained by segmenting the mean TD values over 2912 10-2 VFs in end-stage glaucoma with the median value of the mean TD at all test locations. **(C)** The original mean TD values over all 10-2 VFs in end-stage glaucoma. All VFs are plotted in right eye format. Reproduced from Wang *et al.*[31]

Hood *et al.* analyzed the association between macular structure and the 10-2 VF in eyes with normal 24-2 VF findings and recognized 2 distinct zones associated with the central VF (discussed in previous chapters).[29] They observed that the inferior temporal zone of 10-2 VF is particularly less vulnerable to glaucomatous damage and the remaining region of 10-2 VF is more vulnerable to damage (Figs. 11-2 last row, 11-3). The Hood model has been authenticated for advanced and early glaucoma.

6. A study on central VF loss patterns and their shifts in advanced glaucoma

A retrospective cohort study provided a quantitative characterization and classification of central VF patterns and their shifts of central VF loss in advanced glaucoma.[31] The study analyzed a total of 2912 reliable 10-2 VFs of 1103 eyes from 1010 patients with advanced glaucoma (Figs. 11-3, 11-4). They included patients with advanced glaucoma having 24-2 VFs with an MD of -22 dB or less. In this study, an MD value of -22dB was considered as the cutoff point for end-stage glaucoma. The 10-2 VFs with test dates on or after any 24-2 VFs with an MD of -22 dB or less were included for data analyses.

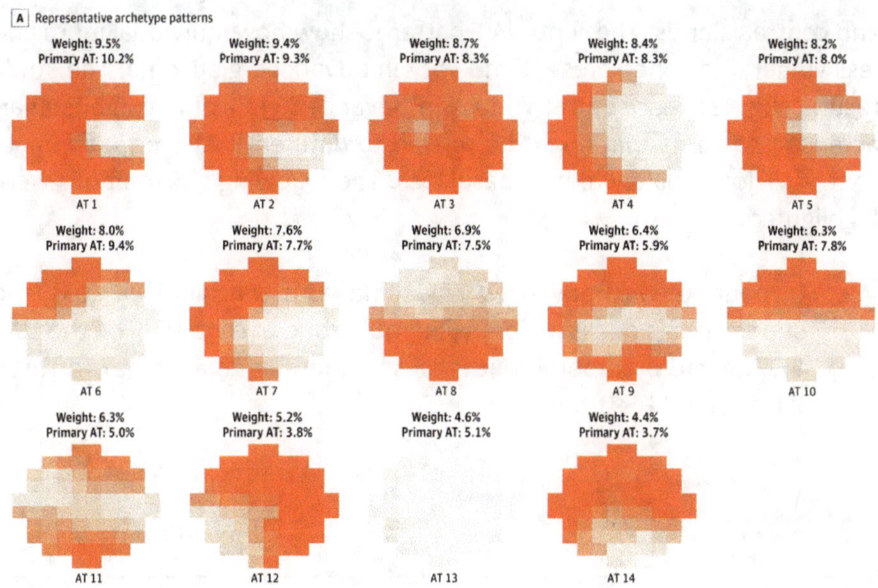

Fig. 11-4. The 14 central 10-2 VF patterns in end-stage glaucoma. The 14 archetypes include nearly intact central vision (archetype 13), temporal-sparing loss (archetypes 1, 2, and 5), hemifield loss (archetypes 8 and 10), inferonasal quadrant sparing (archetype 12), central island loss (archetype 9 and 11), nasal loss (archetypes 4, 6, and 7), nearly total loss (archetype 14), and total loss (archetype 3). Reproduced from Wang *et al.*[31]

The TD values were used as primary inputs for assessing the VF loss pattern by archetypal analysis (Fig. 11-4). Central VF patterns were determined by an artificial intelligence algorithm termed archetypal analysis. Longitudinal analyses were performed to investigate whether the development of CVFDs mostly affects specific vulnerability zones.

First, the unsupervised artificial intelligence method of archetypal analysis was applied to characterize the spatial patterns of 10-2 VF loss in advanced glaucoma. Next, the study compared the 10-2 VF loss patterns with the more vulnerable and less vulnerable zones proposed by the Hood model. Finally, they quantified the development of 10-2 VF defects over time for the eyes with the patterns that preserved the entire less vulnerable zone at baseline.

This study quantitatively determined the representative central VF loss patterns in advanced glaucoma, including patterns of nearly intact VF, nearly total loss, total loss, temporal sparing, quadrant sparing, nasal loss, and central islands. The central VF patterns show how individual more and less vulnerable zones present and vary in advanced glaucoma. The study results suggest that central VF loss in advanced glaucoma exhibits characteristic patterns that might be related to different subtypes, and initial central VF loss is likely to be a nasal loss. The following observations were highlighted.

- In patients with advanced glaucoma with central visual loss, the superonasal zone is a more vulnerable zone of central VF on the 10-2 VF. The inferotemporal zone is a less vulnerable zone of the central VF (Figs. 11-2, 11-5A).

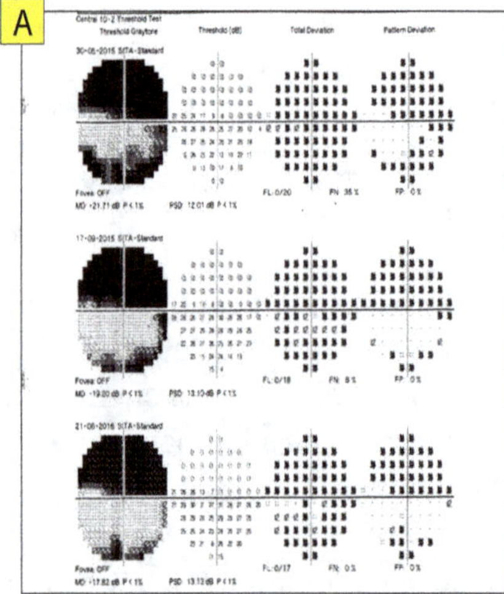
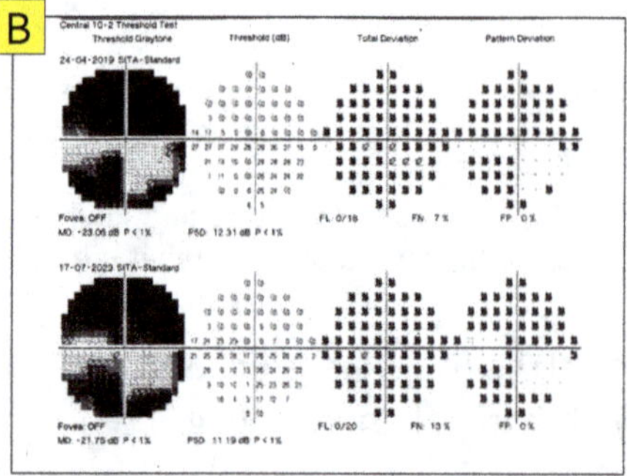

Fig. 11-5. Overview printout of a 10-2 VF of the left eye of an 80-year-old OAG patient with advanced-stage glaucoma and best-corrected visual acuity of 20/80 (logMAR +0.6). The patient is non-hypertensive, non-diabetic, and has no macular pathology. He has bilateral pseudophakia and has minimum glaucomatous damage in his right eye. IOP is 12 mmHg in the left eye, well controlled with maximal medical therapy, and shows very little progression of VF loss over a little more than 8 years. **(A)** The 3 fields shown in this overview printout show a negligible change in MD and PSD over an 8-year period from 2015 to 2023 in the patient's left-eye 10-2 VF. In 2015, MD was -21.7 dB and PSD 12 dB on the 10-2 VF; in July 2023, MD was -21.7 dB and PSD 11.1 dB on the 10-2 VF. **(B)** However, a recent deterioration is noticed within the central 5° region in the last 10-2 VF (2023) and new defects occur in the less vulnerable zone from the temporal side.

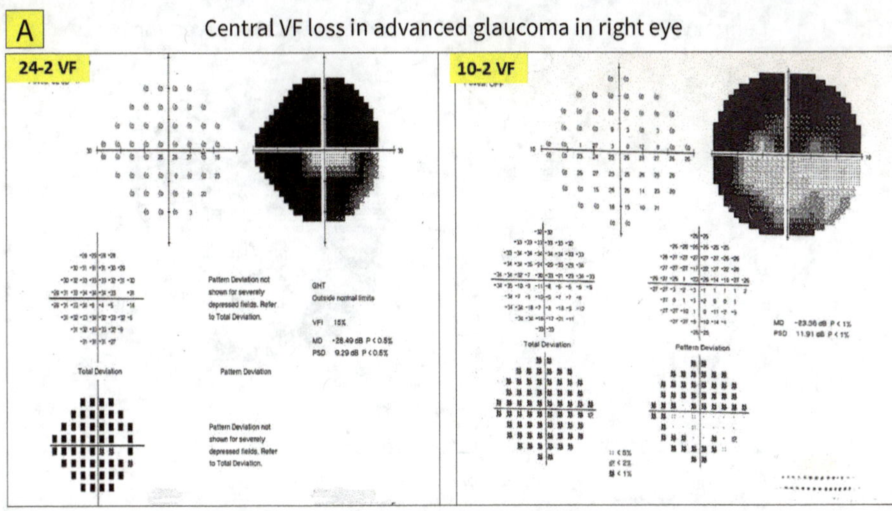

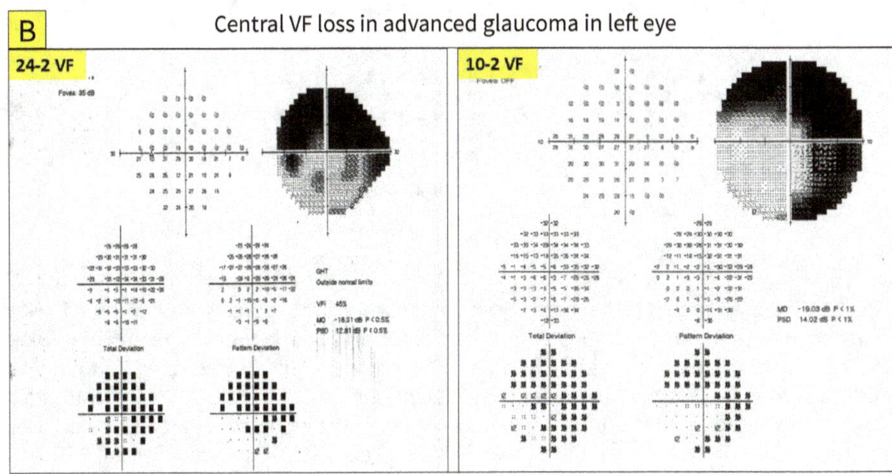

Fig. 11-6. The effect of trabeculectomy combined with phacoemulsification on the central VF in an advanced glaucomatous eye. Findings on 10-VF before and after the surgical intervention are documented here. This 70-year-old patient was diagnosed with bilateral NTG. The patient's 24-2 and 10-2 VF show advanced glaucomatous loss bilaterally, more severe in the right eye (MD -28.49 dB) than in the left eye (MD -18.31 dB) on 24-2 VF. The right eye had cataract and a best-corrected visual acuity of 20/70 (+0.6 logMAR), while the best-corrected visual acuity in the left eye was 20/25 (+0.1 logMAR). IOP was 8 mmHg and 10 mmHg in the right and left eye, respectively, on maximal medical therapy. His VF condition had been monitored to this advanced stage of glaucoma by 10-2 VF testing as 24-2 VF testing provides little information when only the central island of vision remains. **(A)** Advanced VF loss on both 24-2 and 10-2 VF in his right eye. A part of the inferonasal and the less vulnerable inferotemporal zone of the central VF was unaffected. **(B)** VF defects in his left eye on 24-2 and 10-2 VF.

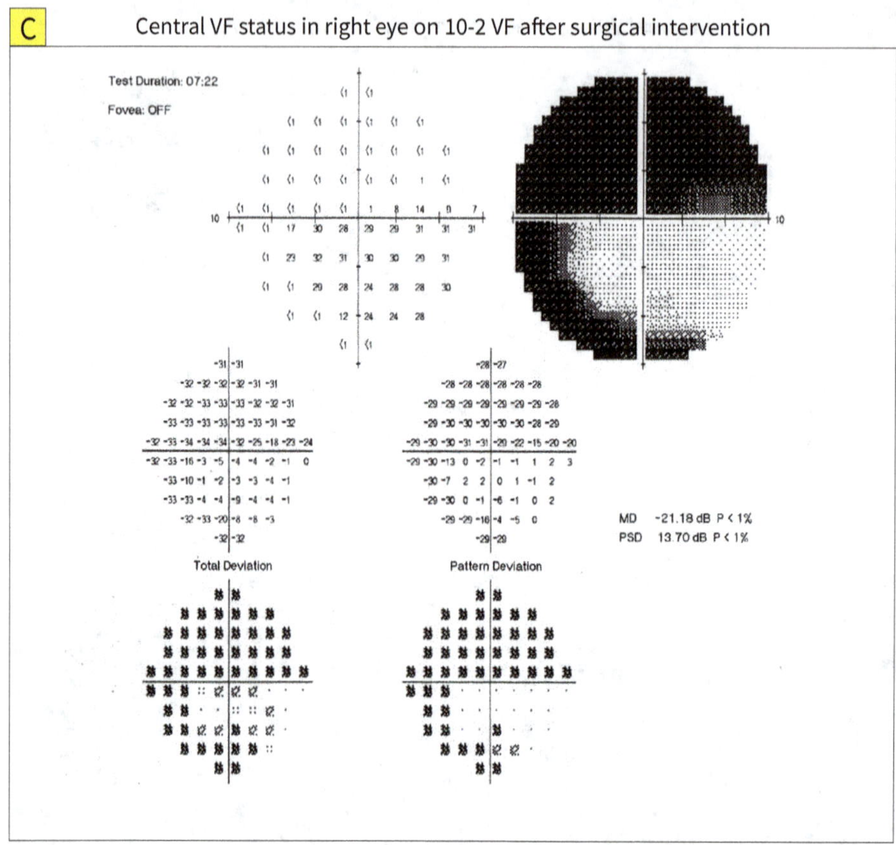

Fig. 11-6. Continued. **(C)** The patient had undergone trabeculectomy combined with phacoemulsification and intraocular lens implantation in the right eye in February 2023. The central VF status in his right eye on 10-2 VF remained unaffected after 3 months of this procedure and his best-corrected visual acuity improved to 20/30 (0.2 logMAR) after surgery. The preoperative values for MD and PSD in the right eye were -23.36 dB and 11.91dB, respectively. Postoperatively, MD was -21.18 dB (slight improvement) and PSD was 13.70 dB (a bit worse).

- VF damage in more vulnerable zones can take different forms. They specifically mentioned the 14 central VF loss patterns (Fig. 11-4). The most common defects in the central VF are: temporal sparing patterns, followed by mostly nasal loss, hemifield loss, central island, total loss, nearly intact field, inferonasal quadrant sparing, and nearly total loss. Initial central VF loss is likely to be a nasal loss, and 1 specific type of nasal loss is likely to develop into a total loss.

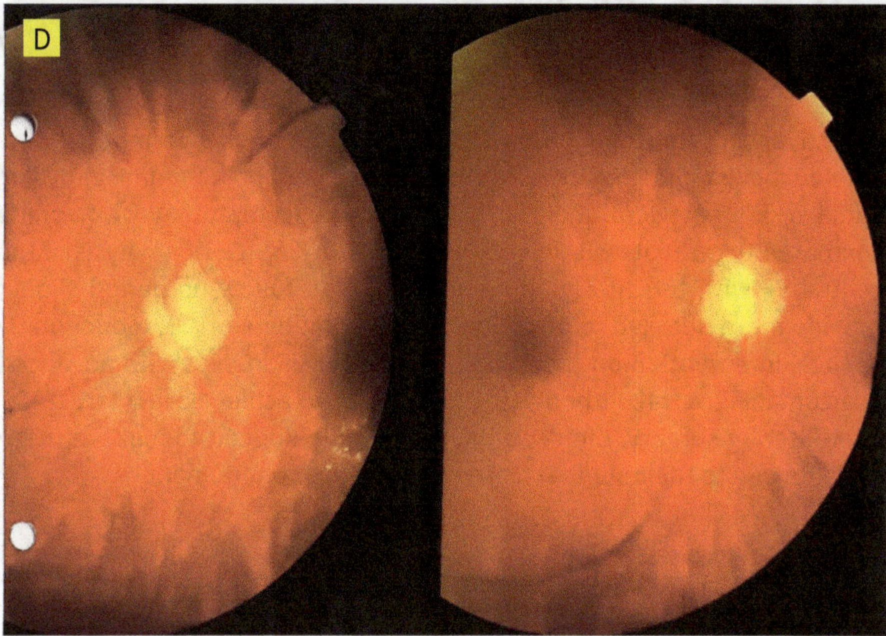

Fig. 11-6. Continued. **(D)** Advanced glaucomatous cupping in both eyes, more pronounced in the right eye than the left eye. This case did not report any occurrences of the wipe-out phenomenon in the 3-month postoperative follow-up after the combined procedure.

- Among the 14 representative patterns, 7 patterns lost specific areas of the more vulnerable zone, whereas only 2 patterns were subject to visual loss in the less vulnerable zone (Fig. 11-3B).
- On 1-year and 2-year follow-ups, new defects mostly occur in the more vulnerable zone.
- A notable finding was that the initial encroachments on an intact central VF at follow-up in end-stage glaucoma tended to take the form of nasal loss patterns that are similar to the known nasal step patterns in early glaucoma development detected by 24-2 VF.

7. Central 10° VF change following filtration surgery in advanced glaucoma

The Advanced Glaucoma Intervention Study demonstrated that patients with advanced glaucoma who achieved a lower IOP (< 14 mmHg) during initial treatment were unlikely to develop glaucomatous VF worsening compared to patients with higher levels of IOP (Fig. 11-1).[7] Analysis of the central VF with the 10-2 program and a longer follow-up period should provide more detailed information about the effects of IOP reduction by surgical intervention on the remaining central VF in eyes with advanced glaucoma (Fig. 11-4). Although it is important to achieve a low target IOP after filtering surgery, the decision is especially difficult to make in these patients due to the potential risk of a "wipe-out" phenomenon.

8. Wipe-out phenomenon following filtration surgery in advanced glaucoma

A number of studies have pointed out the wipe-out phenomenon of irreversible and immediate sudden reduction of visual acuity without any apparent cause after filtering surgery in patients with advanced glaucoma with small residual visual fields.[32] Nonetheless, the actual frequency of this phenomenon is controversial.

The effect of filtration surgery in advanced glaucoma has been extensively studied and the findings have divided investigators into 2 opposite camps. One group points to the danger of performing this surgical procedure on the advanced glaucoma population and warn patients about it.[33] The other group suggests that the risk is minimal or non-existent.[34] This discrepancy in the incidence of wipe-out is probably an outcome of confusions about its definition as well as due to technological advances in surgery. Many studies have recorded macular edema, cataract, and other causes related to sudden visual loss after filtration surgery in advanced glaucoma patients. The loss of vision in some patients with advanced stage was probably wrongly labeled as the wipe-out phenomenon. Moreover, studies reporting a high rate of wipe-out are old studies performed more than a decade ago.

				1	2				
	3	4	5	6	7	8			
	9	10	11	12	13	14	15	16	
	17	18	19	20	21	22	23	24	
25	26	27	28	<u>29</u>	<u>30</u>	31	32	33	34
35	36	37	38	<u>39</u>	<u>40</u>	41	42	43	44
	45	46	47	48	49	50	51	52	
	53	54	55	56	57	58	59	60	
	61	62	63	64	65	66			
			67	68					

Fig. 11-7. Number of VF test locations of the 10-2 program **(right eye)**. Underlined numbers indicate test locations included in the point-wise analysis. Reproduced from Fujishiro *et al.*[36]

A study evaluated the effect of trabeculectomy with mitomycin C on visual acuity and VFs in patients with advanced-stage glaucoma during the immediate postoperative period and assessed the risk of sudden visual loss.[34] The inclusion criterion was a preoperative VF score over 16 as per the grading recommended by the Advanced Glaucoma Intervention Study.[7] The main outcome measures were change in: best-corrected visual acuity, MD of the VF test, number of points among the 4 central VF points with a sensitivity less than 5 dB, and mean sensitivity of the 4 central VF points after surgery (Fig. 11-7). This study did not report any occurrences of the wipe-out phenomenon in postoperative eyes after being followed for 3 months after filtration surgery. In a separate study, investigators evaluated the risk of the wipe-out phenomenon following non-penetrating deep sclerectomy in eyes with advanced-stage glaucoma within the first 6 months postoperative period.[35] Likewise, they did not record any occurrences of the wipe-out phenomenon in the postoperative period. Similarly, Figure 11-6 presents the unaltered status of the central VF in an advanced glaucomatous eye 3 months after the combined procedure (author's unpublished data).

Another study investigated in detail the outcome of trabeculectomy on the central VF in 27 OAG patients with advanced VF damage for 12 months postoperatively using the HFA 10-2 program. The inclusion criteria of the study were (1) raised and normal IOP in OAG eyes; (2) absence of any coexisting ocular or systemic disorders (*e.g.*, cataract); (3) 3 or more reproducible VF test results taken every 6 months with the HFA 10-2 SITA Standard or Full Threshold program before the trabeculectomy, and mean TD of the 10-2 program of ≤ −20 dB and MD of the 30-2 program of ≤ −18 dB preoperative test performed within 1 month before surgery; (4) preoperative best-corrected visual acuity ≥ 40/200 and foveal threshold ≥ 10 dB.[36] TD in each of the 4 test locations closer to fixation (TD_{29}, TD_{30}, TD_{39}, and TD_{40}) were used for the analyses. This study observed that subjects' eyes showed neither any deterioration of visual acuity to 20/200 or less, nor any loss of central VF.

TD values in the central 10-2 program test locations (Fig. 11-7) showed no significant change in that period, but a clinically significant decrease in best-corrected visual acuity without apparent causes was found in only 4% of eyes at 12 months after the surgery.

There is speculation that macular splitting could be another risk factor of the wipe-out phenomenon. Macular splitting is defined as the mean TD value of 2 adjacent test locations of the central 4 test locations in the upper or lower hemifields (TD^{29} and TD^{30}, or TD^{39} and TD^{40}) worse than -20 dB and that of the other 2 locations better than -10 dB. This study observed that 18% of eyes had macular splitting; however, none of them had > 2 lines of deterioration in best-corrected visual acuity at 12 months after surgery. Their findings suggest that trabeculectomy resulted in hardly any change in the central 10° VF. However, a significant decrease in best-corrected visual acuity without apparent cause might occur in approximately 5% of the cases.

References

1.   Social Security Administration, Office of Disability. Disability evaluation under Social Security: 2.00 special senses and speech–adult Vol 2018. Available from: https://www.ssa.gov/disability/professionals/bluebook/2.00-SpecialSensesandSpeech-Adult.htm#203.

2.   Saunders LJ, Russell RA, Kirwan JF, McNaught AI, Crabb DP. Examining visual field loss in patients in glaucoma clinics during their predicted remaining lifetime. Invest Ophthalmol Vis Sci. 2014;55(1):102-109. https://doi.org/10.1167/iovs.13-13006

3.   Foulsham WS, Fu L, Tatham AJ. Prior rates of visual field loss and lifetime risk of blindness in glaucomatous patients undergoing trabeculectomy. Eye (Lond). 2015;29(10):1353-1359. https://doi.org/10.1038/eye.2015.156

4.   Mills RP, Budenz DL, Lee PP, et al. Categorizing the stage of glaucoma from pre-diagnosis to end-stage disease. Am J Ophthalmol 2006; 141: 24-30. https://doi.org/10.1016/j.ajo.2005.07.044

5.   Heijl A, Patella VM, Bengtsson B. The Field Analyzer Primer: Excellent Perimetry, 5th edition. Carl Zeiss Meditec; 2021.

6.   Lee SH, Joiner DB, Tsamis E, et al. Optical coherence tomography circle scans can be used to study many eyes with advanced glaucoma. Ophthalmol Glaucoma.2019;2(3):130-135. https://doi.org/10.1016/j.ogla.2019.02.004

7.   King AJ, Fernie G, Azuara-Blanco A, et al. Treatment of Advanced Glaucoma Study: a multicentre randomised controlled trial comparing primary medical treatment with primary trabeculectomy for people with newly diagnosed advanced glaucoma-study protocol. Br J Ophthalmol. 2018 Jul;102(7):922-928. https://doi.org/10.1136/bjophthalmol-2017-310902

8.   Hodapp E, Parrish RK, Anderson DR. Clinical decisions in glaucoma. Mosby: St Louis C.V.; 1993.

9.   Joussen AM. Graefe's archive for clinical and experimental surgery-170th anniversary. Graefes Arch Clin Exp Ophthalmol. 2024 Mar;262(3):673-675. https://doi.org/10.1007/s00417-023-06358-w.

10.   Varma R, Ying-Lai M, Francis BA, et al.; Los Angeles Latino Eye Study Group. Prevalence of open-angle glaucoma and ocular hypertension in Latinos: the Los Angeles Latino Eye Study. Ophthalmology. 2004;111:1439-1448. https://doi.org/10.1016/j.ophtha.2004.01.025

11.   King AJ, Stead RE, Rotchford AP. Treating patients presenting with advanced glaucoma-should we reconsider current practice? Br J Ophthalmol. 2011;95:1185-1192. https://doi.org/10.1136/bjo.2010.188128

12.   Leighton P, Lonsdale A, Tildsley J, King A. The willingness of patients presenting with advanced glaucoma to participate in a trial comparing primary medical vs primary surgical treatment. Eye. 2012;26:300-306. https://doi.org/10.1038/eye.2011.279

13.   Traverso C, Walt J, Kelly S, et al. Direct costs of glaucoma and severity of the disease: a multinational long term study of resource utilisation in Europe. Br J Ophthalmol. 2005;89: 1245-1249. https://doi.org/10.1136/bjo.2005.067355

14. Fiscella RG, Lee J, Davis EJ, Walt J. Cost of illness of glaucoma. Pharmacoeconomics. 2009;27:189-198. https://doi.org/10.2165/00019053-200927030-00002

15. Lee PP, Walt JG, Doyle JJ, et al. A multicenter, retrospective pilot study of resource use and costs associated with severity of disease in glaucoma. Arch Ophthalmol. 2006;124:12-19 https://doi.org/10.1001/archopht.124.1.12

16. Chakravarti T. The Association of Socioeconomic Status with Severity of Glaucoma and the Impacts of Both Factors on the Costs of Glaucoma Medications: A Cross-Sectional Study in West Bengal, India. J Ocul Pharmacol Ther. 2018 Jul/Aug;34(6):442-451. https://doi.org/10.1089/jop.2017.0135

17. Lee JM, Cirineo N, Ramanathan M, et al. Performance of the visual field index in glaucoma patients with moderately advanced visual field loss. Am J Ophthalmol. 2014;157:39-43. https://doi.org/10.1016/j.ajo.2013.09.003

18. Medeiros FA, Lisboa R, Weinreb RN, Girkin CA, Liebmann JM, Zangwill LM. A combined index of structure and function for staging glaucomatous damage. Arch Ophthalmol. 2012;130(5):E1-10. https://doi.org/10.1001/archophthalmol.2012.827

19. Zangwill LM, Williams J, Berry CC, Knauer S, Weinreb RN. A comparison of optical coherence tomography and retinal nerve fiber layer photography for detection of nerve fiber layer damage in glaucoma. Ophthalmology. 2000;107(7):1309-1315. https://doi.org/10.1016/S0161-6420(00)00168-8

20. de Moraes CG, Liebmann JM, Medeiros FA, Weinreb RN. Management of advanced glaucoma: Characterization and monitoring. Surv Ophthalmol. 2016;61(5):597-615. https://doi.org/10.1016/j.survophthal.2016.03.006

21. Junoy Montolio FG, Wesselink C, Jansonius NM. Persistence, spatial distribution and implications for progression detection of blind parts of the visual field in glaucoma: A clinical cohort study. PLoS One. 2012;7(7):e14211. https://doi.org/10.1371/journal.pone.0041211

22. Mwanza JC, Budenz DL, Warren JL, et al. Retinal nerve fibre layer thickness floor and corresponding functional loss in glaucoma. Br J Ophthalmol. 2015;99(6):732-737. https://doi.org/10.1136/bjophthalmol-2014-305745

23. Rao HL, Begum VU, Khadka D, Mandal AK, Senthil S, Garudadri CS. Comparing glaucoma progression on 24-2 and 10-2 visual field examinations. PLoS One. 2015 May 15;10(5):e0127233. https://doi.org/10.1371/journal.pone.0127233

24. Park SC, Kung Y, Su D, et al. Parafoveal scotoma progression in glaucoma: Humphrey 10-2 versus 24-2 visual field analysis. Ophthalmology. 2013;120:1546-1550. https://doi.org/10.1016/j.ophtha.2013.01.045

25. Bengtsson B, Heijl A. A visual field index for calculation of glaucoma rate of progression. Am J Ophthalmol. 2008;145(2):343-353. https://doi.org/10.1016/j.ajo.2007.09.038

26. Gardiner SK, Demirel S. Detecting Change Using Standard Global Perimetric Indices in Glaucoma. Am J Ophthalmol. 2017;176:148-156. https://doi.org/10.1016/j.ajo.2017.01.013

27. Rao HL, Kumar AU, Babu JG, Senthil S, Garudadri CS. Relationship between severity of visual field loss at presentation and rate of visual field progression in glaucoma. Ophthalmology. 2011 Feb;118(2):249-53. https://doi.org/10.1016/j.ophtha.2010.05.027

28. Miki A, Okazaki T, Weinreb RN, et al. Evaluating Visual Field Progression in Advanced Glaucoma Using Trend Analysis of Targeted Mean Total Deviation. J Glaucoma. 2022 Apr 1;31(4):235-241. https://doi.org/10.1097/IJG.0000000000001985

29. Hood DC, Raza AS, de Moraes CG, Johnson CA, Liebmann JM, Ritch R. The Nature of Macular Damage in Glaucoma as Revealed by Averaging Optical Coherence Tomography Data. Transl Vis Sci Technol. 2012 May 25;1(1):3. https://doi.org/10.1167/tvst.1.1.3

30. Hood DC. Improving our understanding, and detection, of glaucomatous damage: An approach based upon optical coherence tomography (OCT). Prog Retin Eye Res. 2017 Mar;57:46-75. https://doi.org/10.1016/j.preteyeres.2016.12.002

31. Wang M, Tichelaar J, Pasquale LR, et al. Characterization of Central Visual Field Loss in End-stage Glaucoma by Unsupervised Artificial Intelligence. JAMA Ophthalmol. 2020 Feb 1;138(2):190-198. https://doi.org/10.1001/jamaophthalmol.2019.5413

32. Aggarwal SP, Hendeles S. Risk of sudden visual loss following trabeculectomy in advanced primary open-angle glaucoma. Br J Ophthalmol. 1986 Feb;70(2):97-9. https://doi.org/10.1136/bjo.70.2.97

33. Kolker AE. Visual prognosis in advanced glaucoma: a comparison of medical and surgical therapy for retention of vision in 101 eyes with advanced glaucoma. Trans Am Ophthalmol Soc. 1977;75:539-55.

34. Topouzis F, Tranos P, Koskosas A, et al. Risk of sudden visual loss following filtration surgery in end-stage glaucoma. Am J Ophthalmol. 2005 Oct;140(4):661-6. https://doi.org/10.1016/j.ajo.2005.04.016

35. Leleu I, Penaud B, Blumen-Ohana E, Rodallec T, Adam R, Laplace O, Akesbi J, Nordmann JP. Risk assessment of sudden visual loss following non-penetrating deep sclerectomy in severe and end-stage glaucoma. Eye (Lond). 2019 Jun;33(6):902-909. https://doi.org/10.1038/s41433-019-0336-z

36. Fujishiro T, Mayama C, Aihara M, Tomidokoro A, Araie M. Central 10-degree visual field change following trabeculectomy in advanced open-angle glaucoma. Eye (Lond). 2011 Jul;25(7):866-71. https://doi.org/10.1038/eye.2011.74

Appendix

Caution against labelling individuals as having pre-perimetric glaucoma

Subsection 11 of Chapter 6 of this book discusses Retinal Nerve Fiber Layer Optical Texture Analysis (ROTA) and the 10-2 VF assessment in glaucoma. This subsection references a study[1] that emphasizes the significance of using VF tests with higher sampling density, particularly over the central 18°, such as the 10-2 and 24-2C tests. Additionally, the study cautions against labelling individuals as having pre-perimetric glaucoma without considering the spatial relationship between VF stimulus projections and RNFL defects. This appendix addresses an important issue regarding the inconsistent definition of pre-perimetric glaucoma. It is crucial to consider this inconsistency before labelling any patient as having pre-perimetric glaucoma.

1. Perimetric glaucoma and pre-perimetric glaucoma

The diagnosis of glaucoma is based on structural damage, such as glaucomatous optic neuropathy or loss of the RNFL, combined with functional VF loss as measured by SAP. Again, categorizing glaucomatous damage into appropriate stages improves disease management. Previous studies indicate that structural changes may be detectable before functional changes in glaucoma.[2,3]

Weinreb *et al.* comment that "with current technology, detection of structural defects generally precedes detectable functional defects in glaucoma patients while functional defects can precede structural defects in some patients…".[4] Structural tests, which compare results to normative data, often reveal statistically significant glaucomatous changes earlier than functional tests. However, this is primarily due to the greater variability associated with functional tests.[4]

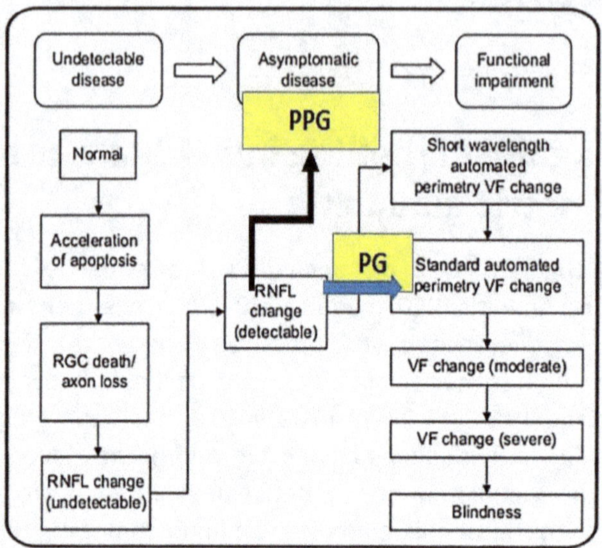

Fig. 1. Glaucoma continuum. PG: perimetric glaucoma PPG: pre-perimetric glaucoma. Reproduced from Weinreb *et al.*[5]

Based on these observations, clinicians and researchers have categorized the progression of glaucoma into 2 distinct stages (Fig. 1):

- **Stage 1** is the **pre-perimetric glaucoma** stage, which is characterized by no functional defects on SAP.
- **Stage 2** is the **perimetric glaucoma** stage, which is characterized by functional impairment on SAP.

2. Definitions of pre-perimetric glaucoma vary significantly: a literature review

An abstract based on a yet unpublished literature review presented at the 2023 World Glaucoma Congress[6] found that the definition of pre-perimetric glaucoma varies significantly due to the absence of standard guidelines. This review had 2 major aims: to determine the prescribed guidelines for defining perimetric glaucoma and pre-perimetric glaucoma using SAP and to identify the differences between the guidelines for perimetric glaucoma and pre-perimetric glaucoma through a systematic review of the reported data on pre-perimetric glaucoma.

This literature review analyzed 36 peer-reviewed articles from PubMed published between 1999 and 2022 based on specific criteria.[7-18] Only prospective studies with "pre-perimetric glaucoma" in their titles were included, while those lacking clear definitions of perimetric glaucoma and pre-perimetric glaucoma were excluded. Due to the variability in study parameters, a meta-analysis was not feasible. The review categorized the guidelines for defining perimetric glaucoma and pre-perimetric glaucoma into 5 groups:
1.   Anderson-Patella Criteria:[19] The-gold standard for defining perimetric glaucoma VF.
2.   Non-specific criteria: Where no specific guideline was mentioned.
3.   Different criteria: Any guideline not matching the existing guidelines.
4.   Cluster criteria:[20] Guidelines based on cluster analysis on Octopus perimetry.
5.   ISGEO Criteria:[21] Characteristics of glaucomatous VF defects.

2.1. Definitions of pre-perimetric glaucoma and perimetric glaucoma

Pre-perimetric glaucoma VFs can be defined as VFs taken before the diagnosis of manifest glaucoma as defined by Anderson-Patella criteria (see Chapter 4, Fig. 4-6).[19] The review found that only 47.2% of studies adhered to Anderson-Patella criteria,[19] which is regarded as the gold standard for defining perimetric glaucoma VF. Of this 47.2%, 43% applied only 1 criterion, while 57% applied all 3 Anderson-Patella criteria.

The majority of the studies utilized other guidelines than Anderson-Patella criteria. Specifically, 36.1% followed alternative guidelines (*e.g.*, 12% followed Budenz's *Atlas of visual fields*[22] to identify perimetric glaucoma VFs), 5.5% used the ISGEO classification, and 8.3% adhered to non-specific guidelines. Among clinicians, 91.4% preferred the Humphrey perimeter over the Octopus perimeter for VF testing. Regarding the indices used, the GHT Outside Normal Limits was the most frequently chosen (63.6%) for developing different guidelines, followed by MD and PSD, both selected by 50% of the studies. Notably, 74% of the research papers did not apply the repeatability factor to confirm glaucomatous VF defects.

2.2. The inconsistent definition of pre-perimetric glaucoma

According to this review:

- Fewer than 50% of clinicians and researchers adhere to the prescribed guidelines for defining perimetric glaucoma and pre-perimetric glaucoma and differentiating between the two.
- Additionally, the implementation of these guidelines is inconsistent and varies significantly among practitioners.
- The repeatability factor, which is essential for confirming glaucomatous VF defects, is often overlooked.
- There are no universally accepted guidelines for defining perimetric glaucoma and pre-perimetric glaucoma in clinical practice and research.
- In glaucoma patients, the detection of structural defects generally precedes detectable functional defects, which is related to the inconsistent definition of pre-perimetric glaucoma and the greater variability associated with functional tests.

2.3 Major challenges of reaching a consensus for defining perimetric glaucoma and pre-perimetric glaucoma

- Wide variability in the guidelines.
- Non-uniformity in the implementation of Anderson-Patella criteria.
- Poor consensus on confirming the reproducibility of glaucomatous VF defects.
- Lack of consistency among conditions for framing structural criteria in defining pre-perimetric glaucoma.
- Poor detection of earliest glaucomatous VF defects by HFA 30-2/24-2 test grid with points 6° apart (see Chapters 4 and 6).

References

1. Leung CKS, Guo PY, Lam AKN. Retinal Nerve Fiber Layer Optical Texture Analysis: Involvement of the Papillomacular Bundle and Papillofoveal Bundle in Early Glaucoma. Ophthalmology. 2022 Sep;129(9):1043-1055. https://doi.org/10.1016/j.ophtha.2022.04.012
2. Wollstein G, Kagemann L, Bilonick RA, et al. Retinal nerve fibre layer and visual function loss in glaucoma: the tipping point. Br J Ophthalmol. 2012;96:47–52. https://doi.org/10.1136/bjo.2010.196907

3. Kerrigan-Baumrind LA, Quigley HA, Pease ME, Kerrigan DF, Mitchell RS. Number of ganglion cells in glaucoma eyes compared with threshold visual field tests in the same persons. Invest Ophthalmol Vis Sci. 2000;41:741–748.

4. Weinreb RN, Garway-Heath DF, Leung C, Medeiros FA,Liebmann JM. Structure Function. Diagnosis of Primary Open Angle Glaucoma: WGA Consensus Series-10. Kugler Publications; Amsterdam: 2017. p. 90–127.

5. Weinreb RN, Friedman DS, Fechtner RD, et al. Risk assessment in the management of patients with ocular hypertension. Am J Ophthalmol. 2004 Sep;138(3):458-67. https://doi.org/10.1016/j.ajo.2004.04.054

6. Chakravarti T. The Definition of Preperimetric Glaucoma Varies a Lot as There Are No Standard Guidelines: A Systematic Review. Abstract WGCABS-429 presented at the 10th World Glaucoma Congress; 2023 June 28-July 1; Rome Italy.

7. Asaoka R, Murata H, Iwase A, Araie M. Detecting Preperimetric Glaucoma with Standard Automated Perimetry Using a Deep Learning Classifier. Ophthalmology. 2016 Sep;123(9):1974-80. https://doi.org/10.1016/j.ophtha.2016.05.029

8. Hohberger B, Lucio M, Schlick S, Wollborn A, Hosari S, Mardin C. OCT-angiography: Regional reduced macula microcirculation in ocular hypertensive and pre-perimetric glaucoma patients. PLoS One. 2021 Feb 11;16(2):e0246469. https://doi.org/10.1371/journal.pone.0246469

9. Chen HC, Chou MC, Lee MT, et al. The Diagnostic Value of Pulsar Perimetry, Optical Coherence Tomography, and Optical Coherence Tomography Angiography in Pre-Perimetric and Perimetric Glaucoma. J Clin Med. 2021 Dec 13;10(24):5825. https://doi.org/10.3390/jcm10245825

10. Nakano N, Hangai M, Nakanishi H, et al. Macular ganglion cell layer imaging in preperimetric glaucoma with speckle noise-reduced spectral domain optical coherence tomography. Ophthalmology. 2011 Dec;118(12):2414-26. https://doi.org/10.1016/j.ophtha.2011.06.015

11. Rolle T, Briamonte C, Curto D, Grignolo FM. Ganglion cell complex and retinal nerve fiber layer measured by Fourier-domain optical coherence tomography for early detection of structural damage in patients with preperimetric glaucoma. Clin Ophthalmol. 2011;5:961-9. https://doi.org/10.2147/OPTH.S20249

12. Hirasawa K, Takahashi N, Matsumura K, Kasahara M, Shoji N. Diagnostic capability of Pulsar perimetry in pre-perimetric and early glaucoma. Sci Rep. 2017 Jun 12;7(1):3293. https://doi.org/10.1038/s41598-017-03550-x

13. Sihota R, Shakrawal J, Azad SV, Kamble N, Dada T. Circumpapillary optical coherence tomography angiography differences in perimetrically affected and unaffected hemispheres in primary open-angle glaucoma and the preperimetric fellow eye. Indian J Ophthalmol. 2021 May;69(5):1120-1126. https://doi.org/10.4103/ijo.IJO_1191_20

14. Rao HL, Addepalli UK, Chaudhary S, et al. Ability of different scanning protocols of spectral domain optical coherence tomography to diagnose preperimetric glaucoma. Invest Ophthalmol Vis Sci. 2013 Nov 1; 54(12):7252-7. https://doi.org/10.1167/iovs.13-12731

15. Lee WJ, Na KI, Kim YK, Jeoung JW, Park KH. Diagnostic Ability of Wide-field Retinal Nerve Fiber Layer Maps Using Swept-Source Optical Coherence Tomography for Detection of Preperimetric and Early Perimetric Glaucoma. J Glaucoma. 2017 Jun;26(6):577-585. https://doi.org/10.1097/IJG.0000000000000662

16. Begum VU, Addepalli UK, Yadav RK, et al. Ganglion cell-inner plexiform layer thickness of high-definition optical coherence tomography in perimetric and preperimetric glaucoma. Invest Ophthalmol Vis Sci. 2014 Jul 11; 55(8):4768-75. https://doi.org/10.1167/iovs.14-14598

17. Shiga Y, Aizawa N, Tsuda S, et al. Preperimetric Glaucoma Prospective Study (PPGPS): Predicting Visual Field Progression With Basal Optic Nerve Head Blood Flow in Normotensive PPG Eyes. Transl Vis Sci Technol. 2018 Jan 23; 7(1):11. https://doi.org/10.1167/tvst.7.1.11

18. Orshan D, Tirsi A, Sheha H, et al. Structure-function models for estimating retinal ganglion cell count using steady-state pattern electroretinography and optical coherence tomography in glaucoma suspects and preperimetric glaucoma: an electrophysiological pilot study. Doc Ophthalmol. 2022 Dec;145(3):221-235. https://doi.org/10.1007/s10633-022-09900-z

19. Asman P, Heijl A. Evaluation of methods for automated Hemifield analysis in perimetry. Arch Ophthalmol. 1992;110(6):820-826. https://doi.org/10.1001/archopht.1992.01080180092034

20. Racette L, Fischer M, Bebie H, Holló G, Johnson CA, Matsumoto C. Visual field digest. A guide to perimetry and the Octopus perimeter. 6th ed. Koniz: Haag-Streit AG; 2016.

21. Quigley HA. Number of people with glaucoma worldwide. Br J Ophthalmol. 1996 May;80(5):389-93. https://doi.org/10.1136/bjo.80.5.389

22. Budenz DL. Atlas of visual fields. Philadelphia: Lippincott-Raven; 1997.